EVERY VICTORY COUNTS®

...for Care Partners
Inspiration and Information for Living Well Today as a Parkinson's Care Partner

BY THE DAVIS PHINNEY FOUNDATION

And by leading Parkinson's experts and dozens of care partners who understand what it takes to live well

SECOND EDITION

© 2021, 2023, 2025 Davis Phinney Foundation.

All rights reserved. No part of this publication may be reproduced, stored in a retrieval system or transmitted in any form or by any means, electronic, mechanical, scanning, photocopying, storage or otherwise, without the prior written consent of the Davis Phinney Foundation. Any unauthorized use of the manual or its contents, in whole or in part, is a violation of applicable copyright and/or trademark laws.

Disclaimer:

This manual may contain opinions, advice, information, data, links to third party website addresses, and other materials belonging to third parties. Any and all such uses are for illustrative purposes only and do not necessarily indicate an endorsement of the opinions, advice, information, data, products or services provided by those third parties. The Davis Phinney Foundation does not claim any proprietary right in, or to, any such items as may qualify as copyrights, trademarks or other proprietary marks of third parties. Subject to the foregoing, this manual, including without limitation, any data, text, information, graphics, images and other materials, and the selection and arrangement thereof, are copyrighted materials of the Davis Phinney Foundation ©2010, 2012, 2014, 2016, 2017, 2019, 2021, 2025 ALL RIGHTS RESERVED. Any unauthorized use of the manual is a violation of applicable copyright and/or trademark laws.

Neither the Davis Phinney Foundation, nor any contributor to the manual, is responsible for the content of the opinions, advice, information, data, or third-party websites contained in the manual provided by other parties, or the manner in which any of the foregoing may be used by any party. The Davis Phinney Foundation and each contributor to the manual disclaim any responsibility to any party for any direct, indirect, incidental, reliance, consequential or punitive damages or any other loss or damages, including without limitation, bodily harm, lost profits, expenses or revenue; regardless of whether the Davis Phinney Foundation or any such contributor knew, or ought to have known, of the possibility of any loss or damage arising from the application or use of any opinions, advice, information or data, or visit to a third party's website, referenced in the manual.

Use of this manual is at your own and sole risk. This manual is provided "as is" and any and all express or implied conditions, warranties or representations, including without limitation, any implied warranty or condition of merchantability, fitness for a particular purpose, noninfringement or any warranty or representation in respect to the accuracy or usefulness of information, or any observations that may be derived from such information are disclaimed.

EVERY VICTORY COUNTS

■ TABLE OF CONTENTS

INTRODUCTION

FOREWORD 7

INTRODUCTION 8

YOUR ROADMAP FOR LIVING WELL TODAY AS A PARKINSON'S CARE PARTNER 9

PART ONE: WHAT DOES IT MEAN TO BE A CARE PARTNER?

What's the difference between a care partner and caregiver/carer/caretaker? 11
What is a Parkinson's care team? 11
How can I help my person with Parkinson's build their care team? 15
What kind of care team should I build for myself as a care partner? 15
What role should I play in managing my person's care? 17
How can I take care of myself and my person with Parkinson's? 17
How is the care partner experience different when my person is living with young onset
    Parkinson's (YOPD) instead of later-onset Parkinson's? 19
How can I maintain a strong relationship with my person with Parkinson's? 20
"How can my person with Parkinson's and I keep the lines of communication open?" ... 22
How do I know when I'm taking on too much as a care partner? 23
What's the best way to approach difficult conversations with my person with Parkinson's? 24
I don't want to nag. So how do I encourage my person with Parkinson's without harping
    or nagging? 26
How can I tell if I'm expecting too much/too little from my person with Parkinson's? .. 26
I feel like nobody gets what we're going through. What kind of resources are available for
    Parkinson's care partners? 28
Does Parkinson's progress in a predictable way? It seems like everyone we meet with
    Parkinson's has different symptoms. What should I expect over the next few years? .. 28
I always hear people say that people don't die from Parkinson's; they die with it.
    Is that true? 31
Honestly, I feel angry about my partner's diagnosis. We had so many plans that are now
    slipping through my fingers. How can I be loving and supportive but also honest about
    how I'm feeling? 31
"What was it like when Parkinson's became part of your lives?" 32
"What are some coping strategies I can rely on when I need them?" 35
How can I be an advocate for my person with Parkinson's? 40
"What do I need to know about palliative care for Parkinson's? In what ways can it help?" 41
What does the data say about the role of a care partner? 44

"How can I live well today as a Parkinson's care partner?" 44

PART TWO: CARE PARTNERS AFTER A PARKINSON'S DIAGNOSIS

My partner is newly diagnosed with YOPD. What should we tell our children? 47

"How might my partner's Parkinson's diagnosis impact our family dynamics?" 49

Should I attend physician appointments with my person with Parkinson's? 51

Should I be responsible for organizing (fill in the blank: medical appointments, medication lists, health care directives, etc.)? 51

We have heard countless people talk about how important exercise is for people with Parkinson's, but my person with Parkinson's won't do it. What should I do? How can I get them to exercise? 51

"My person with Parkinson's is hesitant to tell friends and co-workers about their diagnosis. Why might this be?" 56

What should my person with Parkinson's and I know about disclosing their diagnosis at work? 57

"My person with Parkinson's isn't experiencing any burdensome motor symptoms. Should they begin taking medication anyway?" 58

How can I encourage my person with Parkinson's to maintain their independence as symptoms start progressing? 59

My person with Parkinson's is my parent and lives in another state. How can I help? What can I do to stay involved? What's my role? What should I not do? 61

"What is it like to grow up with a parent who has Parkinson's?" 62

My person with Parkinson's lives alone. How can I help? 64

My person with Parkinson's is my spouse. Since their Parkinson's diagnosis, we have not been on the same page in our desire for intimacy. Will this change? What should we do? 65

My person with Parkinson's is experiencing compulsive behaviors. What is happening? .. 66

My person with Parkinson's has more frequent OFF periods than they did a few years ago. How can I help? 71

The last time we saw a movement disorder specialist, they suggested we have conversations about things like living wills, advance directives, etc. That seems so scary and not necessary right now. Why would they suggest that? 74

Is there anything I should think about with respect to our living arrangements now? When's the right time to make these decisions? 76

How can I make sure Parkinson's doesn't become the center of every conversation? ... 77

"My person with Parkinson's has been experiencing depression and/or anxiety for the past ten years, long before their Parkinson's diagnosis. How can I help them manage this symptom?" 78

How do I balance my work and my role as a care partner? 79

When is it time for my person with Parkinson's to stop driving? ... 80

PART THREE: MANAGING THE COMPLICATIONS OF PARKINSON'S

What kind of activities can I expect to do as my person's Parkinson's progresses? ... 84

My person with Parkinson's is so worried about falling that they don't want to leave the house. How can I motivate them to stay connected to our community? ... 84

"How can I make sure our home is safe for my person with advanced Parkinson's?" ... 86

My person with Parkinson's was diagnosed at age 48 and is now 73. They grew up an avid athlete and exercised regularly with Parkinson's until two years ago when they lost the motivation to continue doing so. Their Parkinson's has progressed rapidly in the past few years. How can I help them get back on track? ... 87

My person with Parkinson's has become apathetic about everything. What can/should I do? ... 88

How can I be most helpful during medical appointments? ... 89

My person with Parkinson's is showing signs of cognitive distress. What should I do? ... 89

"How can I respond in a helpful way when I notice my person with Parkinson's is experiencing cognitive problems?" ... 90

"I have heard that as Parkinson's progresses, a person can develop Parkinson's psychosis. What does this look like?" ... 91

I've noticed that my person with Parkinson's seems to be hallucinating, but when I mention it, they deny it. What should I do? ... 92

My person with Parkinson's hallucinates frequently but isn't bothered by them. Is it okay to let it go? ... 93

My person with Parkinson's is having very extreme hallucinations, and I'm scared when they happen. I don't know how to calm them down. What can I do when it's happening? ... 94

In the past year, my person with Parkinson's has begun experiencing delusions and frequently accuses me of having an affair. No amount of denial can convince them otherwise. What can I do? ... 94

How can I manage the emotional toll I'm feeling from my person's Parkinson's disease psychosis? ... 96

I no longer feel like I can support my person with Parkinson's without additional assistance. Where can I go for help? ... 97

My role as a Parkinson's care partner is the most rewarding I have ever had. It is positive in many ways, but it is impacting me in negative ways as well. I am feeling lonely, exhausted, and underappreciated. What can I do? ... 99

What are some of the signs that Parkinson's is progressing to the most advanced stages? ... 99

"How can I stay positive when facing the advanced stages of Parkinson's?" ... 100

How can I help my person with Parkinson's and myself find joy? ... 100

APPENDIX

PARKINSON'S HOME SAFETY TIPS ... 103
PARKINSON'S CARE PARTNERS: REWRITING THE RULEBOOK ... 108
Rulebook Guidelines ... 108
Rules for Yourself ... 109
Safety First ... 110
Communicating with Your Person with Parkinson's ... 111
Communicating with Your Doctor ... 112
Communicating with Friends and Loved Ones ... 113

INDEX ... 115

Introduction

FOREWORD

BY CONNIE CARPENTER PHINNEY

We created this for you—anyone curious about how to better help their friend or family member with Parkinson's—and truly, I hope it helps answer questions and helps you build your strategy for living well. It is an exceptionally valuable tool, filled with input and tips from the medical community and other caregivers.

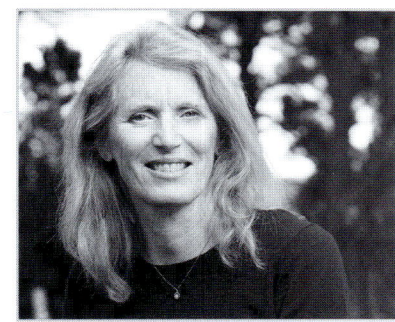

Caring for someone with Parkinson's has brought you to this manual. The fact you are reading this right now means you are showing up for your person and taking steps toward a better understanding of this often unpredictable and sometimes unrelenting disease. Hopefully, reading this will help ease and illuminate your path.

When I speak to caregiver groups, I like to acknowledge at the outset that we dislike Parkinson's. We often say, "I hate Parkinson's," in unison. It feels cleansing to agree on that simple point, right? Now, remind yourself what you love about your person with Parkinson's. Remember, they don't want to be defined by Parkinson's, and neither do you, but it is undeniably a big part of their life and yours. Parkinson's is a game changer but not a game ender.

For those new to this role, a Parkinson's diagnosis can feel like a giant leap into the unknown. It may feel like you are tiptoeing through a minefield. I've been there and know how overwhelming it feels. Some of you, like me, have been in this role a long time (more than two decades for me). We are all learning to navigate and negotiate the changing landscape that is Parkinson's. It can be simultaneously exhausting, confounding, and rewarding. It may surprise you to realize it is the most gratifying job you'll ever tackle.

I hope this manual helps you today and every day. Thanks for showing up.

You can do this!

— CONNIE CARPENTER PHINNEY,
CO-FOUNDER, DAVIS PHINNEY FOUNDATION

INTRODUCTION

Whether you are the spouse, partner, child, parent, sibling, or friend of your person with Parkinson's, you are an invaluable part of their team. Your role as a care partner will evolve throughout the years, but in each stage, it is essential to equip yourself with tools, advice, strategies, and support to ensure that you and your loved one live well. We designed this *Every Victory Counts Manual for Care Partners* to give you just that.

Parkinson's is a complicated and multifaceted condition, and although there are many symptoms, no one person will experience all of them. Learning about the possible symptoms, along with strategies to manage them and actions your person with Parkinson's can take to live well every day, will help both of you. Educate yourself about the spectrum of Parkinson's symptoms and learn which are the most challenging for you and your loved one. Explore trusted websites, books, and articles; watch educational videos; attend support groups and educational events; have conversations with healthcare professionals on your person's medical care team. (And if your person with Parkinson's doesn't have a copy of the sixth edition of the *Every Victory Counts* manual, be sure you order one! Although we designed the manual for people living with Parkinson's, it can also help you understand Parkinson's so you can better support your loved one.)

In our two decades of working to help people live well with Parkinson's, we have met tens of thousands of Parkinson's care partners. With you, we have celebrated, laughed, cried, struggled, and overcome challenges. We have learned strategies to help people with Parkinson's live their best lives. And we have been asked for advice on all aspects of Parkinson's care. Throughout this manual, we will share some of the most frequently asked questions we receive from Parkinson's care partners, with responses from us, from Parkinson's experts, and from Parkinson's care partners. We've designed it to be accessible to all care partners, whether you care for someone young, newly diagnosed, or in the advanced stages of Parkinson's.

Being a Parkinson's care partner means you are special, that someone trusts you enough to ensure their health and safety when they need it most. It is also a role that requires endurance and the ability to take your care just as seriously. If you can balance the caregiving you do for your loved one with the caregiving you do for yourself, you will experience many benefits of being a care partner, including increased health and longevity, purpose, increased confidence, deeper relationships, and more.

YOUR ROADMAP FOR LIVING WELL TODAY AS A PARKINSON'S CARE PARTNER

Even though you love the person you care for, caring for someone with Parkinson's brings physical, emotional, and financial challenges. It's critical to be proactive about your own wellness, just like you encourage your loved one with Parkinson's to be about theirs. Learn about the stress that can come with being a care partner and take steps to limit or avoid factors that lead to burnout. Continually encourage your partner to take an active role in their care; research has shown that when people with Parkinson's have a greater sense of control over their life, everyone's well-being improves. Finally, develop a community of trusted friends, relatives, and other care partners who can provide practical and emotional support.

The key to living well as a care partner is actively choosing to do what will result in your best quality of life. Be informed, be engaged, be connected, and be patient. Each day will bring new challenges and opportunities for positive change. Remember, your daily triumphs, large or small, are worth celebrating: *Every Victory Counts!*

Dear Ken,

Thank you for being my partner in this life. Thank you for seeing me as a woman, a wife, and a mother, not only a person with Parkinson's. You make me a better person, and I could not imagine going through this journey without you. We are stronger together.

Forever, Kat

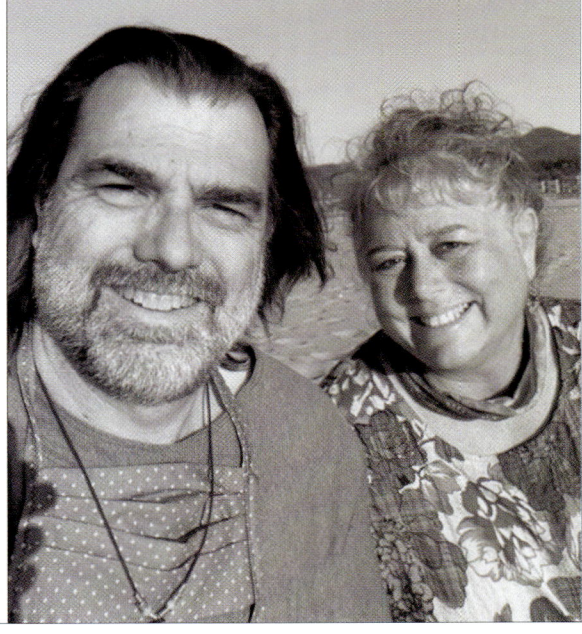

Part One: What Does It Mean to Be a Care Partner?

A Parkinson's care partner is an essential, active member of the care team that supports a person with Parkinson's. Just as Parkinson's affects everyone differently, your role as a care partner will impact you in unique ways. Nonetheless, your journey of living well as a care partner involves many of the same prescriptions we recommend to your loved one living with Parkinson's: take action, stay connected, and get involved.

While many care partners are spouses, care partners can also be children, siblings, parents, and friends. This chapter discusses the types of care partners who support people living with Parkinson's, everyday care partner responsibilities, and ways to give your person with Parkinson's the best care possible. No matter your relationship with your person with Parkinson's, know that you are a vital part of their journey.

WHAT'S THE DIFFERENCE BETWEEN A CARE PARTNER AND CAREGIVER/CARER/CARETAKER?

The difference between a care partner and caregiver is that a care partner is a true partner in care, working closely with their person with Parkinson's in a collaborative, cooperative relationship. Each person in this partnership has an understood role, and there is a shared sense of purpose.

On the other hand, a caregiver provides care for someone who can no longer care for themselves. The relationship is a one-way street. As your loved one living with Parkinson's becomes less independent and more reliant on your care, your role as a care partner may transition to that of a caregiver, or you may get support from professional caregivers to help your person with their increasing needs.

The role of a caregiver is just as essential as that of a care partner. Remember, though, that you do not *have* to do everything alone, and (as we explain in depth in part three of this manual), you do not have to transition into your person's caregiver if doing so does not feel right for you. If that's the case, ask for help, look for other care options, lean on the rest of your person's care team, and recognize your unique role and how it may need to change over time.

WHAT IS A PARKINSON'S CARE TEAM?

Living well with Parkinson's means living well in all aspects of life—physical, mental, social, spiritual. One provider can't possibly treat every part of your person with Parkinson's life, so, ideally, over time, they and you will build a holistic, integrated care team and personalized plan based on their unique symptoms, needs, and goals.

In the beginning, your person's primary care physician and neurologist or movement disorder specialist may be the only two people they need on their care team. However, the team may grow over the years to include anywhere from three to ten or more providers. Everyone is different, and not everyone will need the same types and number of providers. Here are some to consider to give you an idea of the many professionals who can help your person live well.

Note: Before your person with Parkinson's sees their physicians, help them review the worksheets, assessments, and checklists page on our *Every Victory Counts* website. We designed these checklists and worksheets to help people with Parkinson's get the most out of appointments and make sure they communicate with their providers effectively. In addition, as we'll discuss again later in this manual, we encourage you to attend as many appointments with your person and their physicians as possible, for three important reasons: to make sure all the physicians' questions are answered as completely as possible, to be sure the answers are accurate (from your perspective in addition to what your person perceives), and so you can record the conversation to review later.

Neurologist or Movement Disorder Specialist. A neurologist is a physician specializing in the conditions of the nervous system. They can confirm a Parkinson's diagnosis and establish an appropriate treatment plan. A movement disorder specialist (MDS) is a neurologist with additional training in movement disorders. An MDS will most likely be the person on the medical care team who is most familiar with the full spectrum of Parkinson's medications and treatments.

> *Even if they don't think they need one now, encourage your person with Parkinson's to see a movement disorder specialist. They may have much less frequent OFF times if they can add this person to their medical team."*
>
> — CAROLYN RHODES

Primary Care Physician. In addition to your person's MDS or neurologist, their primary care physician (PCP) is a critical part of their team. Your person's PCP will play an essential role in problems unrelated to Parkinson's, monitor their general health, and make sure they stay up to date on preventive medical screenings. A PCP can also help identify potential medication interactions and assist your person with Parkinson's in finding additional specialists if needed.

Nurses. Nurses are potent team members and can be strong liaisons between hospitals, medical offices, and the community, helping create and maintain an integrated approach to care. For many people, nurses provide the first line of access and address many health issues.

EVERY VICTORY COUNTS

If a question or concern is a problem they cannot solve, they know who on the team can. They can also educate people living with Parkinson's and care partners about medication schedules, medical team members, and what to expect throughout a Parkinson's journey.

Neuropsychologist. Neuropsychologists specialize in the relationship between behavior and brain function. Cognitive impairment and behavioral complications such as depression, anxiety, and apathy can be some of the earliest symptoms people with Parkinson's notice, often before receiving an official diagnosis. Most people with Parkinson's will experience these issues at some point. If your person does, a great first step is to be evaluated by a neuropsychologist who specializes in neurological disorders. They can assess your person's thinking skills, including memory, attention, reaction time, language, and visual perception. They will also evaluate your person's emotional functioning. They will combine the results with the rest of your person's medical record to develop a diagnosis and recommendations for improving your person's quality of life.

Social Worker, Counselor, Therapist, or Psychologist. Professionals who focus on emotional health and well-being will be beneficial throughout the Parkinson's journey. Counselors, social workers, therapists, and psychologists are trained to assess emotional difficulties and work with people from all walks of life to promote good mental health. They can help you and your person with Parkinson's cope and stay positive.

Psychiatrist. Psychiatrists are physicians who specialize in mental health. They are qualified to assess both the psychological and physical aspects of mental health issues and prescribe medication. If your person with Parkinson's experiences emotional symptoms such as anxiety, depression, and/or apathy, a psychiatrist can advise them on nonpharmacological management strategies and can also adjust their medication regimen in ways that can help.

Spiritual Advisor/Chaplain. If faith is part of your life, a pastor, chaplain, rabbi, or other spiritual advisors can help you find peace, discover meaning, and accept life changes within the comfort and context of your beliefs.

Physical Therapist. Physical therapy can help your person with Parkinson's improve strength, flexibility, and mobility, and it can also decrease stiffness and pain related to Parkinson's. Many people with Parkinson's don't realize how valuable a physical therapist (PT) can be in the early days (especially if they can find one who specializes in working with people with neurological disorders); however, the people we know who have worked with them consistently have received tremendous value from doing so—both physically and emotionally. When your person begins seeing a PT early after their diagnosis, the PT can teach them exercises that address any current weaknesses, which will allow them to stay stronger and mobile for longer. Also, by getting an assessment early, their PT will see how their Parkinson's is progressing and recommend exercises to address areas that may be getting weaker. If possible, seek out a PT who is trained in movement disorders. Although all PTs receive some training in Parkinson's, those who specialize in neurological physical therapy have a much deeper understanding of Parkinson's and can teach your person exercises specifically designed to help manage Parkinson's symptoms.

Occupational Therapist. Occupational therapy is the only profession that helps people across the lifespan do things they want through therapeutic activities (occupations). Occupational therapy and therapists can help your person with Parkinson's with many everyday activities at work, home, and play, from dressing and eating to overcoming freezing problems to installing and using adaptive equipment.

Speech-Language Pathologist. As Parkinson's progresses, some people have difficulty speaking loudly, pronouncing words, speaking fluidly, and showing facial expression. However, it is possible to improve all these symptoms by working with a speech therapist or speech-language pathologist (SLP). These rehabilitative professionals can also help your person with eating, swallowing issues, saliva management, dry mouth, drool, and more. Developing a relationship with an SLP soon after diagnosis can help prevent acute loss in speech.

Pharmacist. If you and/or your person with Parkinson's see a pharmacist regularly (instead of ordering medications through an online service), they can be a valuable part of your care team. Because they will know all the medications your person takes, those related to Parkinson's and those that are not, your pharmacist will be on the lookout for medication interactions that a primary care physician may not be aware of. Whenever their physician prescribes your person a new medicine, ask your pharmacist (in person or if you order medication online, via phone) if there's anything you need to know about how it might interact with other meds your person is taking. Pharmacists can also advise about crushing pills, splitting doses, and "easy-open" bottles.

Registered Dietician. To find the best nutritional strategy for your person with Parkinson's, see a registered dietician (RD) specializing in working with people with Parkinson's or other neurological disorders. RDs are usually the most qualified health professionals on nutrition and dietetics unless your person's primary care physician, neurologist, or movement disorder specialist specializes in that field.

Dentist, Dermatologist, and Eye Care Professional. Preventive care is important for everyone, and because people with Parkinson's are more susceptible to melanoma and dental problems, it's crucial that they stay up to date on dental and skin screenings and check-ups. Parkinson's can also impact some people's vision, so be sure your person has regular exams with an eye care professional.

Care Partner. That's you! And you are essential to the team and are most likely its captain. As their Parkinson's progresses, your role as the coordinator and manager of their care team will increase.

Family and/or Friends. Your person's family members are also living with Parkinson's and will be critical partners on the team. They can help assemble the rest of the care team and record therapies and outcomes. Look to friends and community as sources of healthy social connectivity and support.

Your Person with Parkinson's. Then, of course, there's your person living with Parkinson's. Your person is the most critical member of the team. Help them think about the role they want to play as the primary team member and continually encourage them to be an active participant in managing their condition and their care team.

HOW CAN I HELP MY PERSON WITH PARKINSON'S BUILD THEIR CARE TEAM?

You and your person with Parkinson's need a support system as you navigate this shared journey. Don't wait to reach out and start adopting a holistic approach. To help your person build a team of providers who can offer expertise in many different areas, become an advocate. Seek out providers who listen, respect your person's input, and with whom your person feels comfortable. If a member of your person's care team is not giving you and your person the time and attentiveness you deserve, find a new care team member. It's perfectly acceptable (and sometimes essential) to fire a physician, rehab specialist, or other healthcare professionals if they aren't meeting your expectations. Being a strong advocate will give your person a solid foundation and help them live well with Parkinson's today and for many years to come.

WHAT KIND OF CARE TEAM SHOULD I BUILD FOR MYSELF AS A CARE PARTNER?

Just as many people can help your person with Parkinson's live well, there are many whom you can add to your care team as you navigate your role as a care partner. Who plays a role in supporting you may change over time, and you may not need the same care team that another care partner does. As you think about who would make a vital part of your team, here are some people to consider:

Financial advisors. The unknowns of any medical condition bring financial questions. Having a trained financial counselor advise you in proactive strategies can reduce confusion and enhance financial peace of mind. Donald L. Haisman, a certified financial planner (CFP) who is living with Parkinson's, says a team of "financial care partners" can assist you and your person with Parkinson's, which could include the following professionals (specific US-based designations in parentheses):

- Accountant (ideally a Certified Public Accountant, CPA)
- Attorney who specializes in estate planning
- Financial planner (ideally a Certified Financial Planner-Professional, CFP)

PART ONE: WHAT DOES IT MEAN TO BE A CARE PARTNER?

- Investment advisor (many times, this is also the CFP)
- Insurance agent (ideally a Certified Life Underwriter, CLU)

Haisman advises you to "share your honest concerns with those professionals on your team; they likely have years of experience assisting families in your situation." He also says that someone on your financial team needs to be the coordinator of all these professionals. "This is very important because these disciplines overlap and contribute to your estate plan. Of the professionals I have suggested, the CFP is most likely to have the overall training, experience, and background to be your coordinator. Often, if you start with a CFP, they can refer you to others, if necessary."

Social Worker, Counselor, Therapist, Psychologist, or Psychiatrist. Just as these professionals can help your person with Parkinson's process and manage emotions and mental health challenges, they can also benefit you. If you need guidance in any aspect of mental health, seek out one or more of these professionals for expert advice and suggestions on coping, resilience, grounding, and much more. We'll take a closer look at various counseling services later in this section.

Spiritual Advisor/Chaplain. Many Parkinson's care partners turn to these advisors for support, guidance, and hope, sometimes within the construct of traditional religions and sometimes through other forms of spiritual expression.

Care partner support group. People we've spoken to who are part of care partner support groups often comment on how important building their community has been. These groups receive emotional support, learn practical advice, and have a safe space to talk about care partner challenges. When you connect with others and bond through shared experiences, you open yourself to greater happiness, growth, and development. Support group members often collaborate on projects, mentor people working in similar fields, become Parkinson's advocates, and build the courage, strength, and resiliency they need to help their people with Parkinson's live well each day.

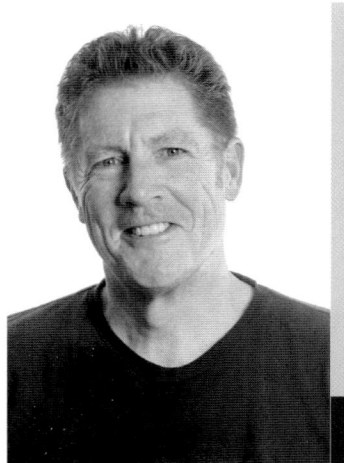

❝ *It's a process of learning and working together. Working with the person in your life with Parkinson's and others as well. It's important to build a Parkinson's village: people with Parkinson's, care partners, friends, and supporters.*"

— **PAT DONAHOO**

Respite care worker. While it might not be in your budget to hire full-time care for your person with Parkinson's, hiring an aide or a respite worker for even an hour a day can make a huge difference in your life. If you're working full time, you might investigate hiring a respite care worker to check in on your person during the day while you're away. If you're not working outside the home, having a respite care worker stop by for even short periods can give you time to devote entirely to yourself—to relax, recharge, exercise, or engage in one of your hobbies. If there's an aspect of caregiving that is especially challenging for you, whether physically or emotionally, hire someone to take it over or ask a good friend or family member to help you out. You don't have to do everything on your own.

Close friends. Now, more than ever, you need trusted friends to turn to for support, love, and fun. The need for these relationships seems obvious; however, when you're helping your person live well with Parkinson's, sometimes tracking medications, going to appointments, exercising, preparing healthy food, and taking care of family take up nearly every minute of your day. Many care partners we've talked to said fun often stays at the bottom of the list. Don't forget to stay connected to your friends and build time into each week to decompress, laugh, and simply have fun with them. Those same care partners said how much their lives improved when they built time for fun, play, and friendships into their day.

You. Take care of yourself first. This is often a challenge when your person with Parkinson's is constantly on the top of your mind and needs a great deal of care; however, you cannot give something you don't have. To love and care for them, you must love and care for yourself. To ease their discomfort and pain, you must be able to ease yours as well. Self-care is not indulgent or selfish. Instead, it is your ticket to living well. And when you live well, you're much better equipped to help them do the same.

WHAT ROLE SHOULD I PLAY IN MANAGING MY PERSON'S CARE?

As we'll discuss later in this manual, the role you'll play in managing or helping manage your person's care will evolve as their Parkinson's changes. No matter what, though, you must communicate often with your loved one to help them understand and accept your concerns and desire to help and support them. Talk about how much you expect or wish to be involved in care. Transitioning from spouse, child, parent, or friend to care partner can change your relationship with your loved one with Parkinson's. Have discussions with your person about expectations.

HOW CAN I TAKE CARE OF MYSELF AND MY PERSON WITH PARKINSON'S?

Know your role and the role of others. Encourage your person with Parkinson's to manage as much as possible and adjust that load as needed. Can they be the manager of their exercise routines? Can they set timers and schedules for taking their medications? Who else can help? Can a friend bring you dinner every Tuesday night? Make a list of the members of your care team and how each can help with your person's day-to-day routines. Teach your person with Parkinson's to ask for and accept care from others early in the game.

> *I have a lot of support from my family and community. It works because I know it's there, but I'm not smothered by it. As people with Parkinson's, we need space to swim and still do things independently!"*
>
> — EDIE ANDERSON

Stay connected. At the Davis Phinney Foundation, we believe that besides medication, the most important ways to live well with Parkinson's are exercise and connection. While social isolation is a rising concern in the general population, it is even more common for people living with chronic illnesses such as Parkinson's. Social isolation's psychological and physical effects can be severe, exacerbating a person's motor and non-motor symptoms, putting them at risk for developing other health problems, increasing their chances of experiencing depression and anxiety, accelerating cognitive decline, and decreasing quality of life. For these reasons and more, it's essential to keep your loved one with Parkinson's connected to your community, friends, and family. You must stay connected as well. Take time to meet friends regularly. Reach out to other care partners and members of the Parkinson's community who understand your challenges and can offer support. Volunteer. Join an exercise, art, music, theater, or other group class. Whatever you enjoy, do it often and stay social.

Consider counseling. One way to take care of yourself and your person with Parkinson's is through counseling. Counseling comes in a variety of forms, from formal psychiatric sessions to self-help books and podcasts. Seeking professional help is a positive, proactive step toward improving your quality of life (and, in turn, being the best care partner you can be).

Unlike a heart-to-heart conversation with a close friend, talking with a professional counselor or therapist can help you explore the foundations of your concerns or worries and learn advice about making positive changes. Like physicians, many therapists have specialties, so finding someone with experience with your unique challenges—whether that is burnout, irritation, relationships, depression, anger, or something else entirely—can be especially helpful.

Counselors can be talk therapists, chaplains, cognitive behavior therapists, social workers, psychiatrists, psychologists, life coaches, or other professionals. As you do when choosing all your healthcare providers, take time to get to know potential counselors and find someone who listens, understands, and supports you.

You can also choose whether you'd like to explore counseling in a one-on-one session or as part of a couple, family, or bigger group.

- Individual Counseling. Many people find it easiest to work through emotional issues by working with a counselor individually. In this setting, you can discuss any concerns you have in a private, one-on-one session.

- Group Counseling. Group counseling can provide a social outlet for individuals who experience common problems. In this type of counseling, individuals with similar problems form a group with a counselor to discuss their problems together. In addition, it is sometimes easier to gain insights and identify positive coping strategies when learned through others' experiences. This type of counseling differs from community support groups in that the counselor helps facilitate the discussion and directs proactive outcomes.

- Relationship and Family Counseling. Parkinson's can be difficult for you as a care partner, your person with Parkinson's, and your family. Many times, when the spouse becomes the care partner, the relationship dynamics change. The goal of relationship counseling is to provide a safe place for communication and honesty. This, in turn, may help to redirect time and energy to the quality of the relationship.

Prioritize self-care. To take care of anyone else, you must first take care of yourself. Taking time away from your care partner responsibilities benefits everyone. Go for a walk or to a yoga class. Read a book. Water your garden. Take a bath. Journal. Watch mindless TV. Take coffee or walking breaks with colleagues during your workday to recharge so you can arrive home energized. Whatever helps you refuel, do it!

Practice forgiveness. There are times in all relationships, especially when one or both people feel tired or frustrated, when something is said in anger or exhaustion. Likewise, there are times in all relationships when someone feels and expresses impatience. Remember this when you react impatiently or unkindly to something your person with Parkinson's says or does. Forgive them when they react in the same manner.

HOW IS THE CARE PARTNER EXPERIENCE DIFFERENT WHEN MY PERSON IS LIVING WITH YOUNG ONSET PARKINSON'S (YOPD) INSTEAD OF LATER-ONSET PARKINSON'S?

YOPD is often (though not always) defined as being diagnosed with Parkinson's when you are younger than 50. The emotional, social, physical, and psychological needs of those diagnosed with YOPD are often different from those diagnosed at an older age. For example, your person with Parkinson's might be soaring in their career, expecting a baby, raising multiple school-age children at home, or getting ready to buy their first house. These concerns are different than those of people who are diagnosed later in life. In addition, although YOPD is characterized by the typical four symptoms of Parkinson's (rigidity, slowness of movement, tremor, and postural instability), the progression of these symptoms is slower. Presenting symptoms also tend to differ for people with YOPD: the most common initial symptoms for YOPD are rigidity and painful cramps. In contrast, the most common initial symptoms for later-onset Parkinson's are tremors and instability while walking.

Given the many differences between YOPD and later-onset Parkinson's, your priorities as a care partner will likely differ from those of partners caring for people diagnosed later in life. Your role may begin and stay for many years in the realm of emotional support. Once people are diagnosed with YOPD, they often struggle with how to share their diagnosis. Due to fear of potential job implications, some choose not to tell their boss or co-workers. Some feel isolated because they don't know anyone else their age with Parkinson's. Some withdraw completely because facing it head-on is too overwhelming. These are all normal responses to hearing the news that you have a chronic and progressive disease; however, if your person with YOPD delays the initiation of appropriate care due to these factors, it can negatively impact their quality of life. (It can negatively impact yours as well; keeping a YOPD diagnosis a secret delays your ability to seek support. Your life has been turned upside-down, too.) For these reasons, it's important to work with your person with YOPD and plan to share their diagnosis in a way that allows both of you to feel comfortable and supported.

In addition, your person may need your encouragement to start a regular exercise program, improve their sleep hygiene, take their medications consistently, connect with others, eat well, and take action to live well every day. Regardless of your person with Parkinson's age, now and at the time of diagnosis, constant communication is essential to being a supportive care partner. Ask your person with YOPD what they need from you and remember that you are their *partner* in care.

HOW CAN I MAINTAIN A STRONG RELATIONSHIP WITH MY PERSON WITH PARKINSON'S?

Positive relationships and supportive environments play a significant role when it comes to facing adversity. The better our relationships, the better our health, outlook on life, and belief in our self-efficacy and resilience. When we have stable relationships, we feel less stress while facing adversity and are more capable of overcoming challenges.

Although Parkinson's can affect relationships over time, for many people, these impacts can be positive. Couples and families who cope most successfully tend to understand and prepare together for the challenges of Parkinson's. Coming together in times of adversity can sometimes strengthen relationships, which can undoubtedly be true after the diagnosis of Parkinson's. Take this moment as an opportunity to examine your life and decide what's most important to you. Prioritizing your close relationships can be vital during times of change and uncertainty.

The keys to maintaining any strong relationship are communication and understanding. Learn how Parkinson's can affect your person's voice, facial expressions, and mood, for all of these can affect how you "see" them when they communicate with you. For example, if your loved one suffers from depression or apathy, it may appear to you that they just don't care. Parkinson's often blunts a person's facial expressions; a condition referred to as facial masking. If your person experiences facial masking, you may not be able to tell what they're feeling based on outward cues. Your person may also experience softer, more monotone speech, which can sometimes cause care partners and friends and family to assume the person is uninterested in what's happening around them, even if the opposite is true. Don't assume that your person feels a certain way based on how they look and know that sometimes you may just need to allow extra time for them to respond and resist speaking for them when they are slow to reply.

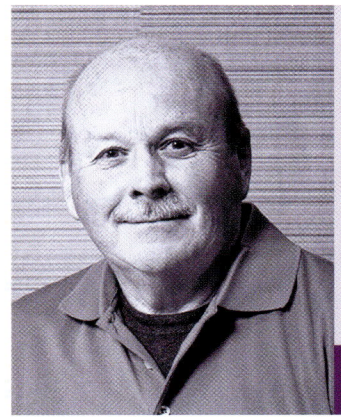

" *The biggest thing I've learned is that you have to separate the person you married who is living with Parkinson's from the issues you may have had with your spouse all along.*"

— SCOTT ANDERSON

Many members of your person's integrated care team can be instrumental in helping with these communication concerns. For example, a speech-language pathologist can help your loved one manage voice and language concerns, facial masking, and other communication symptoms. (Two of the main goals of speech therapy include improving a person's ability to communicate effectively and helping them to enhance communication in social interactions.) If your person experiences depression, anxiety, and/or apathy, a mental health specialist can advise on therapies and medications that can help. (To learn more about Parkinson's and mental health symptoms, check out Chapter 4 of the *Every Victory Counts* **manual** for people living with Parkinson's.)

Reminding yourself and letting others know about some of the symptoms, either seen or unseen, that your person is experiencing can also foster greater understanding and stronger relationships for everyone involved.

"How can my person with Parkinson's and I keep the lines of communication open?"

By Nancy Bivins, LMSW

One of the most critical components of a good Parkinson's journey is maintaining an ongoing, open dialogue. Communicate regularly with each other about your concerns and perspectives. The renowned social scientist Virginia Satir developed a template to guide these kinds of conversations for couples called "The Daily Temperature Reading." She offers five communication tools:

1. Share appreciation for the other person. The more specific this communication, the better. Instead of saying, "You're a good help," say, "Thank you so much for helping me weed the garden."

2. Share new information. This could be a change in plans, gossip, a fear, something of interest, or anything else that helps your loved one keep up with what is going on in your life.

3. Ask inviting, non-judgmental questions instead of assuming you know the answer. For example, ask, "Why did you choose not to go to lunch with Bob?" instead of making a statement like, "You should have gone to lunch with Bob instead of isolating yourself."

4. Pair a complaint with a suggestion. For instance, "Yesterday you said X, but I would appreciate it if you would instead say Y." Listen to the words but also listen to the emotions behind the words. If the two are incongruent, address the feeling you perceive: "You seem sad."

5. Share wishes, hopes, and dreams. Invite each other into your wishes, hopes, and dreams for this day, this year, and your long-term future. Talk to each other, share, and remember that it is healthy for both of you to keep a balance between giving and receiving.

About Nancy Bivins

Nancy Bivins received her Master of Social Work degree from Arizona State University. She serves seniors and people living with disabilities. Eight years ago, she joined the community outreach team at the Muhammad Ali Parkinson Center in Phoenix. This position has allowed her to meet people living with Parkinson's and their families and provide encouragement, support, and information as they face the challenge of living well.

HOW DO I KNOW WHEN I'M TAKING ON TOO MUCH AS A CARE PARTNER?

As a Parkinson's care partner, it's easy to become so focused on your person with Parkinson's that you put your needs on the back burner. This can lead to care partner burnout or, in its extreme, compassion fatigue, where you become overwhelmed physically, emotionally, spiritually, and socially to the point where you're unable to care for yourself or others.

After working closely with care partners for almost two decades, we've identified some of the most common signs of caregiver burnout:

- Moods change on a dime—you feel furious one minute and sad and helpless the next
- Lack of energy
- Overwhelming fatigue
- Sleep problems (too much or too little)
- Trouble concentrating
- Changes in eating habits, appetite, and weight
- Feeling blue, irritable, helpless, and possibly depressed
- Difficulty completing everyday household tasks
- Excessive coffee drinking or increase in unhealthy habits such as smoking, drinking, or abusing prescription medications
- Role confusion and uncertainty on how to be both a care partner and a spouse
- Loss of interest in activities you once enjoyed
- Neglect of your own physical needs
- Lack of exercise
- Feeling that caregiving is controlling your life and that it's the only thing you have time for
- Not letting anyone else help you and needing to control every aspect of care
- Becoming unusually impatient, irritable, argumentative, and maybe even rough with the person you're caring for
- Anxiety about the future
- Placing unreasonable expectations on yourself and beating yourself up if you fail to meet them
- Headaches, stomach aches, and other physical problems
- Lowered resistance to illness—you catch every bug that comes your way
- Withdrawal from friends, family, and other loved ones
- Feelings of wanting to hurt yourself or the person you're caring for

PART ONE: WHAT DOES IT MEAN TO BE A CARE PARTNER?

- Emotional and physical exhaustion
- Losing control physically or emotionally

The good news is that by paying attention to these signs, you'll know if you're headed toward care partner burnout, and you'll be able to take action to avoid it. Throughout this manual, we'll explore many strategies to help you do this. But, for now, here's a list of three actions you can begin *today* to avoid care partner burnout.

#1 - Join a support group. One of the most helpful actions many of the care partners we've worked with have taken has been joining a care partner support group. These groups give you the chance to meet others who share similar experiences, make friends, and remind you that you're not alone. Need help finding one? Head to our website at **dpf.org** and connect with one of our Ambassadors, who can help you find resources in your community.

> *We tend to connect when we're really struggling. You realize that somebody is going through the exact same thing you are, with kids at home, or a husband leaving his job, etc. Lots of similarities. The opportunity to connect with others in similar situations when you need it, whether in a regular support group or online, is really good."*
>
> — **SHERYL**

#2 - Talk it out. It may be uncomfortable to talk to your person with Parkinson's about your experience as a care partner, but open communication is critical to your relationship. Ask your person with Parkinson's what is most helpful to them, ask them what they wish you did more, and let them know about any of the struggles or challenges you're having. Give your person ample time to express their wishes, needs, and challenges. Many people with Parkinson's feel guilty about the role their care partner has been forced into; ask your person if they feel this way, and if they do, talk through those emotions. The more open and honest you are with each other, the less likely you will be to take it all on yourself and go down the path of resentment or burnout.

#3 - Take care of yourself. To love and care for your person with Parkinson's, you must love and care for yourself. Self-care is your ticket to living well as a care partner.

WHAT'S THE BEST WAY TO APPROACH DIFFICULT CONVERSATIONS WITH MY PERSON WITH PARKINSON'S?

Timing is one of the most important things to consider before beginning a difficult conversation. For example, initiating a difficult conversation when you're in the heat of the moment or when your person with Parkinson's is OFF is a recipe for disaster. If you begin the conversation when your person is feeling overly tired or when their medications aren't working optimally, they will likely not be fully present for the discussion. So, if you know the conversation will be difficult, why not do it when you are both feeling ON and open?

Here are a few ways you can let your person know you'd like to talk to them about something:

- I'd like to discuss something with you that I think will help us navigate X more effectively.
- I'd like to talk to you about X, but first, I'd like to get your perspective.
- I'm feeling frustrated about X. Do you have a few minutes to talk about it this afternoon?
- I think we have different perceptions about X. I'd love to know what you think about it. Can we set aside some time tonight to talk about it?
- I'd like to talk about X because I think we may have different ideas about X. Can we talk about it over lunch tomorrow?

Once you have scheduled your time to discuss the issue, prepare for the conversation. Consider the following:

- What do you hope to accomplish by talking about this issue?
- What would be the ideal outcome?
- What assumptions are you making about your person with Parkinson's regarding this issue or how you think they will respond?
- Why is this conversation going to be difficult for you? What role do you have in identifying it as difficult?
- What needs or fears do you have about the impending conversation?
- What role have you played, and what role do you think your person has played, in the situation leading up to the conversation?

Once you get into the conversation, remember that you will feed off each other's energy. Take a deep breath to center yourself as needed and notice if you are having trouble regulating your emotions. If you are, express that to your person with Parkinson's. Keep that openness throughout. And during the conversation, consider the following:

- Can you be more curious than correct?
- Can you listen more and talk less?
- Can you put yourself in their shoes?
- Can you seek to understand and acknowledge them rather than defending your view?
- Can you state your case/opinion without minimizing theirs?
- Can you solve the problem together?
- Can you be okay with the conversation not going your way?

PART ONE: WHAT DOES IT MEAN TO BE A CARE PARTNER?

Know that you may not arrive at the expected outcome right away. As we mentioned earlier, practice forgiveness and patience with one another, and remember that you're both doing the best you can.

I DON'T WANT TO NAG. SO HOW DO I ENCOURAGE MY PERSON WITH PARKINSON'S WITHOUT HARPING OR NAGGING?

Remember that you and your loved one with Parkinson's are a team, and communication is vital. One very effective way to reduce the inclination to nag is to schedule weekly check-ins when you give each other permission to communicate your wants and needs. During these short sessions, ask your person with Parkinson's what worked and what didn't over the week. Then, tell them what did and didn't work for you. Finally, use this time to talk about frustrations, communication misses, and your goals or expectations for the week.

We tend to nag someone when we believe they should do something they either don't want to do or said they wanted to do but don't do. For example, maybe your person with Parkinson's knows they should exercise, but they don't like it. You also know it's an essential ingredient if they want to live well with Parkinson's; so, you get frustrated that they aren't doing it, which causes you to ask them about it every day. This makes sense. You know it's good for them, and you want to support or encourage them to do it. However, it's also important to remember that they are in charge of their life and just because they have Parkinson's, it typically doesn't mean that they have lost their ability to make choices for themselves. You can communicate your concerns during your weekly check-ins, but then it's time to let go and give them the gift of captaining their own ship.

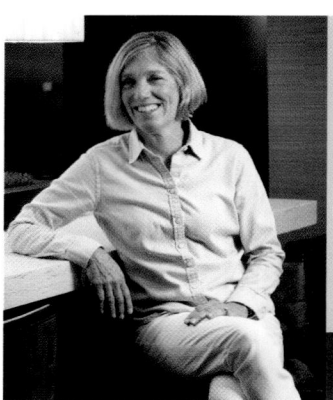

" Finding the line between being a care partner and being a nag is something I have to think about. I try not to be motherly or add pressure but to be supportive. I help when I know he needs the help, but I give him the dignity of doing things independently."

— NANCY HOVEY

HOW CAN I TELL IF I'M EXPECTING TOO MUCH/TOO LITTLE FROM MY PERSON WITH PARKINSON'S?

This is something care partners struggle with a lot. On the one hand, they want to be as helpful as possible, but on the other hand, they want to help their person maintain independence. Keep in mind that not all struggle is bad. Yes, tasks, activities of daily living, and life or house chores may get done much more quickly if you do them yourself; however, if you take over everything, it may take purpose and meaning away from your person and lead them to feel useless or resentful. For example, suppose your person doesn't feel like exercising because they are tired or feeling slow and know that exercise will feel "hard," and you don't encourage them to get out there anyway. In that case, you may avert an argument about it and soothe them, but they will suffer in the long term because they will miss out on all the benefits exercise brings.

There's a sweet spot that takes time and experience to figure out. Just know that it is okay for your person to be challenged, and it's okay for you to encourage their independence. The more they can stay fully engaged in their life, the more they will build self-efficacy and resilience. And the more they continue to do on their own, the more agency and control they will feel, not just about their life but about living with Parkinson's.

Having said that, pay attention to your person. Maybe they have less energy and feel extra tired because they haven't been sleeping or have started a new medication. Or maybe they overdid it the day before in their exercise class. Maybe their fatigue has nothing to do with Parkinson's, and their lack of desire to do anything is a sign that something else is wrong. Pay attention. Notice. And keep the lines of communication open. The better you understand your person with Parkinson's, the better you can set expectations.

> *It's possible that I have the best care partner a person could hope for. Dan is amazingly attentive to my every need, sometimes before I am even aware of it. His challenge is to know when he is being too helpful. I need to be able to feel as though I am as self-sufficient as is feasible."*
>
> — PATTI BURNETT

Dear J., my husband, best friend, and care partner,

Thank you for the support you continue to give me day after day, year after year. I know you want to indulge my hobbies when you ask if I'm ready to go to the craft store or bookstore. I know you mean only the best when you ask, "did you take your meds?" for the third time that day. I know you want me to be strong when you say, "I'm going out to pump the bike tires; see you in a minute," even though I just said I didn't feel like exercising.

»

> I also know that when you make the bed or start fixing a meal without saying anything, your actions speak volumes. Thank you for all that you say and do as we navigate this journey together.
>
> Lorraine

I FEEL LIKE NOBODY GETS WHAT WE'RE GOING THROUGH. WHAT KIND OF RESOURCES ARE AVAILABLE FOR PARKINSON'S CARE PARTNERS?

Often as a care partner to someone with Parkinson's, you need a solution to a problem, but you don't have hours on end to search for it. We're here to help. This manual is one way; another is our continually-updated collection of care partner resources on our ⌕ *Every Victory Counts* **website**. There, you can find worksheets, checklists, app recommendations, and numerous nuggets of wisdom from people who have been caring for someone with Parkinson's for long enough to know how valuable time is and how time-consuming and emotionally and physically taxing being a care partner can be when you don't have the formal training or resources you need. You can also pick up your complimentary digital copy of ✎ **The Parkinson's Care Partner Rulebook**, a collaboration between Connie Carpenter Phinney and the Davis Phinney Foundation that can help you write your own rulebook for living well with Parkinson's, empowering you and your person with Parkinson's to achieve optimal health and well-being. Connie emphasizes that the rulebook is ever-evolving, just as Parkinson's is, and encourages you to be patient, be flexible, and don't be afraid to change the rules as you go.

DOES PARKINSON'S PROGRESS IN A PREDICTABLE WAY? IT SEEMS LIKE EVERYONE WE MEET WITH PARKINSON'S HAS DIFFERENT SYMPTOMS. WHAT SHOULD I EXPECT OVER THE NEXT FEW YEARS?

Everyone's experience with Parkinson's is different, so much so that anticipating its progression can be frustrating. Physicians rarely try to predict the exact course of someone's Parkinson's or how severe or mild their symptoms will be. Each person's symptoms change at different rates and present different variations. Sometimes things change for the better in one area, but a new symptom will crop up elsewhere. Age of onset and overall health can also influence the progression of Parkinson's.

There are, however, similarities most people with Parkinson's experience over time. Symptoms typically evolve slowly. Often, the person with Parkinson's may not be aware of a change in mobility, cognition, or other symptoms until someone else points it out. In the beginning stages of Parkinson's, symptoms such as tremor, slowness, and rigidity typically begin on one side of the body, then spread to the other side over time. Walking, speech, or swallowing problems can occur, too, though these symptoms usually progress slowly over many years. For most people, balance problems occur in later stages, leading to concerns about falls and serious injuries.

Here's an example to make this a bit more concrete. You may have seen your person with Parkinson's complete some tests in their physician's office. A common test for people with Parkinson's is simply tapping the index finger together with the thumb repeatedly. For many people with Parkinson's, the ability to do this action declines rapidly; some people can only manage five or ten taps of the fingers. Try it yourself and notice how you can (likely) tap your thumb and forefinger together for a while, probably without decline. Now, take a moment to consider how that decline in function might translate to other parts of their body and mind. It's a cumulative slowing of function that occurs with Parkinson's—in the muscles, in the gut, and in the brain. Couple that with disrupted sleep, fatigue, mood changes, and more, and you can start to imagine the challenges that your person with Parkinson's has on a daily (and nightly) basis.

How your person's Parkinson's progresses and the different motor and non-motor symptoms they experience will be unique to them. In general, however, the stages of Parkinson's tend to look something like this:

PRE-DIAGNOSIS

There are many non-motor symptoms of Parkinson's that people experience long before they notice motor symptoms; however, it's usually only in hindsight that they realize those were the first signs of Parkinson's. Some of those symptoms include:

- Sleep challenges and disturbances
- Constipation
- Depression and anxiety
- Loss of smell (hyposmia)
- Dizziness and fainting

EARLY STAGE

- Generalized fatigue
- Symptoms on one side of the body
- Decreased arm swing on one side when walking
- Decreased stride length
- Dragging a foot while walking
- Scuffing toes, especially when tired

- Change in leg coordination when cycling or running
- Sense of muscle fatigue or heaviness in arm or leg on one side of the body
- Difficulty completing repetitive movements due to muscle fatigue
- Trouble with hand coordination, especially on one side. This is often apparent doing tasks that use both hands, like shampooing hair
- Reduced range of motion in the shoulder, shoulder pain, or frozen shoulder
- Mask-like face or change in facial expression (hypomimia)
- Decreased or small handwriting (micrographia)

MID STAGE

- Symptoms on both sides of the body
- Soft speech (hypophonia)
- Mild swallowing problems, such as difficulty swallowing pills
- Flexed or bent posture and shuffling gait
- Motor fluctuations and dyskinesia
- Cognitive impairment
- Gastrointestinal dysfunction
- Urinary problems
- Sexual problems
- Pain
- Facial masking

ADVANCED STAGE

- Postural instability with balance problems and falls
- Walking problems, with increased shuffling, freezing of gait, and festination (an involuntary quickening of gait)
- Significant speech and swallowing problems
- Drooling
- Rigidity in the neck and trunk parts of the body
- Vision problems
- Shortness of breath
- Increased cognitive impairment

As your person moves through the different stages of Parkinson's, help them reach out to current and new members of their care team who can help them manage changing symptoms. Remind them, too, that there are many actions they can take to live well and maintain a high quality of life at every stage. Advocate for your person during appointments, ask for referrals, and encourage them to try new exercises and therapies.

I ALWAYS HEAR PEOPLE SAY THAT PEOPLE DON'T DIE FROM PARKINSON'S; THEY DIE WITH IT. IS THAT TRUE?

This is a phrase that people often cite, but it's not as black-and-white as this. The reality is many people will die due to complications that arise because of Parkinson's. For example, falls and pneumonia are two significant causes of death for those with Parkinson's. When people fall and require surgery, that can lead to infections, issues with anesthesia, blood clotting, etc. When a person with Parkinson's gets pneumonia, their difficulty with swallowing and coughing can make it impossible for them to expel mucous, leading to aspiration and death. So, while Parkinson's was not the direct cause of death, the complications of Parkinson's were.

HONESTLY, I FEEL ANGRY ABOUT MY PARTNER'S DIAGNOSIS. WE HAD SO MANY PLANS THAT ARE NOW SLIPPING THROUGH MY FINGERS. HOW CAN I BE LOVING AND SUPPORTIVE BUT ALSO HONEST ABOUT HOW I'M FEELING?

First, it is 100% okay to feel angry. It is 100% okay to feel sad. It is 100% okay to feel grief. It is 100% okay to feel confused, or frustrated, or lost, or whatever you are feeling. Science supports the idea that genuinely *feeling* your feelings by taking the time to notice them, accept them, sit with them, and give them space can make you a healthier and happier person (even when those feelings may seem negative and overwhelming). You are likely grieving the diagnosis just as your person with Parkinson's is. Know that this is a stage almost all people with Parkinson's and their care partners experience, and one that you should acknowledge, process, and allow to take place.

When you're a care partner, your life can seem like nothing but intense emotions, especially in the beginning. Acknowledging and working with your emotions is a key to mental health. Counseling, which we discussed earlier in this manual, can be a very effective way to learn how to notice, process, accept, and work with your emotions. For more on coping strategies and mental wellness, be sure to see the response below by social worker Jessica Shurer.

Consider thinking about your life with Parkinson's as a designer would think of a project. When designers encounter a problem, rather than *think* their way forward, they *build* it. They build it by reframing the problem and then acting. Your design plan is yours to make. The plans that you had before diagnosis may still be possible with time, or your plans may change and be better than you could imagine. Allowing for the impossible may seem like dreaming, but you might surprise yourself with the result when you take action toward your dreams and goals.

PART ONE: WHAT DOES IT MEAN TO BE A CARE PARTNER?

"What was it like when Parkinson's became part of your lives?"

By Connie Carpenter Phinney, MS

Parkinson's entered our lives when our kids were small, and Davis' career was thriving. But truly, it had been lurking and provoking us for years. Fatigue was the primary early symptom that affected our marriage and family, but Davis unwittingly was dealing with various symptoms. I remember nagging him to pick up his feet when he walked because he stumbled a lot. His voice softened, and TV producers asked him to modulate his voice better, but he couldn't seem to do it. The tremor emerged in the spring of 2000, and that is what finally got him to the doctor—or in his case, to many doctors.

Diagnosis is traumatic. And for a while, it felt like the bottom had fallen out of his world. Max Testa, his cycling team doctor from Italy, remarked that it would take him two years to adjust and adapt to this new challenge. He was right. But the neurologist who told him that he'd feel "as good as ever" was wrong. So, you get mixed messages even from physicians, and in the end, how you respond to the diagnosis depends on where you are in your life.

Once we settled into the new life—post-Parkinson's diagnosis—we did realize how lucky we were in one sense. Davis stopped traveling. He had been on the road working somewhere between 75 and 100 days of the year. This was far less compared to his previous life as a cyclist when he was away more than 150 days a year. But it was a lot for the kids and me. So, Parkinson's gave us one treasure: We got Davis back. He is a gifted father. It would have been a shame for him to miss so many fun years with the kids.

My dad told me an interesting thing one night when we were talking about the course of his life. He said that when my mom was diagnosed with multiple sclerosis, he lost his ambition. He wondered aloud if that was a bad thing. I asked him, "In what regard?" And he said that he was content with his family business and never had the desire to risk growing it. He thought maybe he could have made more of his life. I told him that he was the best dad imaginable and that I was so grateful for that. While I knew he worked hard, he put his family first, and caring for us kids and my mom was his best work.

For me, when pressed, I can tell you that watching my strong man (Davis) suffer is tough; the diminishment of so many of his strengths is heartbreaking. It is our reality, and we accept it. There's a fine line between giving in and giving up. I think we strive to stay on the high wire every day. Some days, he has to give up some of what he's planned to do, but it's not like throwing in the towel. It's the rest required of an athlete who is preparing for another day. Together we put one foot in front of the other. Some days feel more daunting than others, but we know good days will come.

On a daily basis, the hard part has been keeping Davis tasked. I could do it all, and people who know me can attest to this. If I did do it all, I'd probably start to feel angry and overburdened. I realized that Davis needed to be engaged in his daily life, and if he was going to stay home, he had better contribute. I give him duties and departments—cars, bikes, dishes, for example. Initially, our bike camp business was thriving, and I still needed him to help with that. Physically, when he couldn't manage to ride his bike, he could photograph our clients and provide slide shows or videos of the week-long tours. I learned to parcel out tasks that he could do. Granted, the fog that he often lives in mentally and the weight of Parkinson's on him physically make every day challenging, and often we need to be spontaneous in terms of what he can do, day by day. I find that if we try to share the burden, then each of us feels better.

Perhaps harder still for Davis was life outside of the home. He was uncomfortable, self-conscious, and tended to isolate himself. Going to the store was a chore. Luckily, our daughter, Kelsey, did not mind accompanying him, and her grown-up demeanor at a young age aided us greatly. I have always tried to bring the outside in, where we can control it best and where he is most comfortable. We even remodeled our house to make it more Davis-friendly: calming walls and spaces and comfortable chairs were keys to helping him live better.

Enlisting the kids is important, and both of ours have helped us a lot. How you include your children in the dialogue of Parkinson's is up to you. We've always been honest with our children without overburdening them. That is a line you will have to tread. I think the difficult years for our kids were the med-cycle years, which were very uncomfortable for Davis and tended to make him very moody. In that case, it was especially important to talk about why Dad felt so uncomfortable and how that affected all of us. It's most important for the kids not to have to carry too much of the burden; not easily done if your kids are sensitive but worth the dialogue to make it clear, all the same.

We had the opportunity to live in Italy for three years and make the most of our bike camp business there. It was a good excuse to start fresh and give the kids a chance to learn a foreign language and live outside their culture. It bought us a lot of time to adjust to the disease, as well (we moved there two years post-diagnosis). We all thrived—primarily because we depended on each other so much. The family dynamic was strongest when we were united so closely, and every day was an adventure. Not everyone has this opportunity, but everyone does have the opportunity to rewrite the way they live. Parkinson's can give you a second chance in how you live your life. Surprisingly, Davis' Parkinson's opened doors that would have otherwise stayed closed because of the busy life he led before his diagnosis.

We try not to be defined by Parkinson's. Many things conspire to give me a rich life. Davis' sense of humor and worldview, our active kids, a few close friends, and my close family all give me much more than a safety net. They are the fabric of my life. I'm not always happy

PART ONE: WHAT DOES IT MEAN TO BE A CARE PARTNER?

about the omnipresent weight of Parkinson's, but then, neither is Davis. We didn't ask for Parkinson's to enter our home. It is an unwanted guest here for a long stay. We have made peace with that aspect.

We share many things—love of sports, physical activity, arts, books—and seek out moments of daily awe in nature. Our now adult children give us great joy, and we pay attention to them together. We share the burden of Parkinson's well, talk about it a lot, assess our family and business goals together, and accept with grace both the good and the bad days.

We wake up in the morning expecting a good day. That's where it starts—every day with a touch of optimism. I hope you can try to do that, too.

To my dear, sweet, amazing, life- and care-partner, Connie,

It is impossible for me to appropriately thank you for everything you do and have done for me throughout our 20+ years with Parkinson's, which is roughly half the time that we've been married. I am incredibly fortunate to have you by my side, most especially through the most challenging times. You are always there for me, nurturing and supporting me with your humor and grace, with your patience and understanding, and with your wisdom.

You protect me, both from myself and my own symptom-lead inabilities (and bad habits). You engage me, whether through your invitation to do a yoga routine, take a walk, listen to a podcast, or head out on a bike ride together. Your gentle prods to do my part with the household chores (the Zen of vacuuming!) allows me to contribute. In essence, you keep me moving and thinking.

You are my voice when mine falters. You are my team leader when it comes to my medical care, marshaling whoever is needed in the pursuit of keeping me functioning at my best I try to express my gratitude often. And I do my best to give you the time and space you need for your own projects, which I know is vital for your own well-being. You are an excellent nutritionist.

You challenge me to do more, use my voice, be more present, laugh more, and live with grace. Through your ministrations, I've managed to keep my symptoms mostly in check for all these years.

»

> I appreciate that it's never easy for you, but your unconditional support allows me to wake every morning with the affirmation, I can and will live well today!
>
> With enduring love and gratitude, Davis

"What are some coping strategies I can rely on when I need them?"

By Jessica Shurer, LCSW

Like people with Parkinson's, care partners face changing roles, relationships, and lifestyles throughout the progression of Parkinson's. You may have noticed complex and evolving emotions during these changes and transitions: guilt that you're "not doing a better job," regret about things that happened in the past, sadness related to your loved one's diagnosis, anger at the universe, family members, or even your loved one with Parkinson's. These emotions are a normal and understandable part of the experience. Give yourself space and energy to cope with them.

"*But I'm fine.*"

Perhaps you're thinking, "I'm fine; I don't need coping strategies." No matter how well you're doing, it can still be beneficial to find time for self-care and self-reflection. You might not want anyone to worry about you, or you may feel selfish for bringing attention to your own needs because you're not the one living with Parkinson's. There also can be a stigma around mental wellness and a tendency to believe that going it alone equates to strength. Care partners getting stuck in this perception is very common, often feeling, "No one can do it as I can," or "If I am not here, something will go wrong." This stalwart attitude and refusal to give necessary care and space to yourself can lead to feeling run down and frazzled, which isn't beneficial for anyone.

COPING STRATEGIES TO FOSTER BALANCE AND WELLNESS

There are many coping strategies that Parkinson's care partners consider effective. Here are 12 suggestions you can try to balance your well-being and your partner's needs.

#1 - Check in with yourself.

We tend to ask others how they're doing but forget about ourselves. Doing regular self-check-ins fosters self-awareness. Ask yourself:

- "How am I doing with this?"
- "What has been my attitude towards Parkinson's?"
- "Am I missing out on things that are important to me and that I enjoy?"
- "What would be helpful for me right now?"

When you attend to your own feelings and needs as a *person*, you can do what you need to do as a *care partner*.

#2 - Look for signs of burnout.

Being a care partner can feel overwhelming and leave you feeling down at times, but it can lead to burnout if this becomes the norm. Try to notice if you've been more irritable or angry, socially withdrawn, have had difficulty concentrating, experienced anxiety or depression, missed your own medications or medical appointments, or have had trouble sleeping at night. These are all red flags that the current care situation may not be sustainable. If you notice that your health is compromised, now is the time to make positive changes or reach out for additional help.

#3 - Be your own advocate.

You are the expert when it comes to your care partner experience. As you advocate for your loved one with Parkinson's, remember to stand up for yourself as well. Assert your rights, share your knowledge, determine your goals, recognize your limitations, and negotiate and communicate your needs. You may find that self-advocacy is quite empowering!

#4 - Embrace "me time."

People with Parkinson's and care partners often spend more and more time together as Parkinson's progresses. For some, this can increase intimacy and connection; for others, it can stress the relationship or erode your sense of self. It's critical to carve out time away from Parkinson's when you are the priority, even if those moments are brief.

Carving out time for yourself, of course, is often easier said than done, especially as your person's Parkinson's progresses. If you are among the majority of people without resources to access professional respite care, remember that help does not have to come in a professional form. Talk with family members, friends, neighbors, and community members to see who may be able to step in to help your person with Parkinson's for certain periods and give you time to step away from your care partner responsibilities for a bit. Could a friend come over each Tuesday for a 30-minute visit with your loved one so you can get lost in a book? Does a family member live nearby who could step in for you once or twice a month so you could see a movie with a friend? Ask for help so you can do whatever you need to do to recharge your batteries and return with more energy and a clearer head.

#5 - Ask for help.

What aspects of your support system can you continue to build? What if you need additional assistance down the road? You might worry about being a burden if you ask for help or accept the help offered but remind yourself and your loved one with Parkinson's that you don't have to go it alone. Think of ways that others can help, whether it is taking your dog for a walk on a day when you have too many appointments, hanging out with your person with Parkinson's while you run an errand, or making you dinner during a hectic week of appointments. If you have not done so already, it might be a good time to try a Parkinson's support group. Care partners are often surprised by the relief they feel from meeting other people they can relate to. Learn about other available resources, such as professional in-home care and mental health counseling that may provide additional support now or down the road.

#6 - Laugh.

Life doesn't stop being funny with a Parkinson's diagnosis. Too many of us take ourselves too seriously! Enjoy the humor in the moments life presents and laugh when something silly occurs. It's OK to laugh at the strange situations Parkinson's can sometimes cause, too. Laughing can be cathartic, especially in those awkward moments. It can also be a relief for the person with Parkinson's to share that laughter with you.

#7 - Have an attitude of gratitude.

In your role as a care partner, find time to recognize the silver linings that give you hope and perspective in the more trying times. Reflect on what Parkinson's has made you grateful for, such as your family, or that Parkinson's isn't the diagnosis that you initially feared. Pause to embrace the fond memories you and your partner share. You can even ask yourself what good has come from Parkinson's or what gifts it has given you. Though it may sound strange, many people report receiving the gifts of time, more meaningful relationships, or new beginnings that wouldn't have been possible without Parkinson's.

Like carving out "me time," practicing gratitude can be tricky for some care partners. We often hear from people living with Parkinson's who, after their diagnoses, express their gratitude about discovering new creative talents or finding a new circle of wonderful friends. It can be more challenging for care partners to find that sense of gratitude; after all, Parkinson's isn't something you or your person signed up for. If you feel this way, seek out a support group and/or a mindfulness program to help you learn how to build moments of gratitude into your daily life.

PART ONE: WHAT DOES IT MEAN TO BE A CARE PARTNER?

#8 - Practice communication and find connections.

Adapting to life with Parkinson's is a partnership between you and your loved one, so it's beneficial to remain on the same page. Good communication fosters closeness and connection. Create times to connect and enjoy one another when the focus is not on Parkinson's. Practice open, honest communication about each of your needs, big decisions, and your future together

#9 - Recognize your strengths.

Whether your loved one has been diagnosed with Parkinson's for one month or 25 years, recognize that you are entering new territory and that you are gaining knowledge that will ultimately give you strength. What's given you strength through this period? In what ways have you surprised yourself? What skills have you gained? Davis Phinney calls these acknowledgments "Moments of Victory." Take strength from them and celebrate them!

#10 - Find meaning.

Every experience is a learning opportunity. You may not be conscious of it, but adapting to life with a complex and chronic condition can lead to personal growth. Think about your Parkinson's story and what this journey has meant to you. Many care partners find a sense of purpose in supporting their loved one with Parkinson's. When faced with new challenges and transitions, try to see the big picture and focus on what matters most to you.

#11 - Stay flexible.

A Parkinson's care partner once sent me this quote: "Blessed are the flexible, for they shall not be bent out of shape." Sometimes, when everything else is unpredictable, the only thing that is in your control is the choice to "go with the flow." Care partners who practice resiliency and adapt to changes as they come have an easier time coping with Parkinson's and a more positive overall mindset than those who resist Parkinson's at every turn.

#12 - Be kind to yourself.

It can't be said too often: you are doing the best you can, and that is more than good enough!

About Jessica Shurer

Jessica Shurer, MSW, LCSW is the Director of Patient and Carepartner Advocacy of CurePSP, whose mission and services are dedicated to the awareness, education, care and cure of atypical Parkinsonism diseases—progressive supranuclear palsy, corticobasal degeneration, and multiple system atrophy.

Prior to joining the team at CurePSP in October 2021, she served as the Center Coordinator & Clinical Social Worker of the Movement Disorders Center at the University of North Carolina at Chapel Hill, a Parkinson's Foundation Center of Excellence and CurePSP Center of Care. She had been in this previous position since graduating UNC Chapel Hill with her Master of Social Work in 2012. Her clinical and research interests include the psychosocial needs of navigating neurodegenerative disease, integrated healthcare models, and palliative and end-of-life care.

Dear Sharon, my care partner and partner in life,

You have always been there for me – regardless of the degree of my need for help. For the first eight years after my diagnosis, I didn't feel like I needed much from you, but recently things have changed dramatically. Due to my spinal issues and overall Parkinson's stiffness, you have done most of the bending and twisting I need to avoid. You never seem to tire of helping me button a shirt or lace my shoes before a walk. Whether it's retrieving dropped pills or getting me situated in bed at night, you have done it with patience and grace I could never match. Joining me for all my physician visits has been so important to me and provided that second set of ears that we both agree is so valuable.

I can't adequately express my admiration for the skills you have developed for teaching others about Parkinson's and helping people with Parkinson's who are following a similar path. Your spirit is indomitable, and you have become an active member of the Care Partner Support Group here in Boulder and play a critical role on our support group's planning committee.

It takes time, energy, effort, and commitment to continue hanging in there with me - despite feeling tired, frustrated, overwhelmed at times. This is not what you signed up for when I was diagnosed.

Nevertheless, I couldn't be luckier than to have you in my life.
Rich

PART ONE: WHAT DOES IT MEAN TO BE A CARE PARTNER?

HOW CAN I BE AN ADVOCATE FOR MY PERSON WITH PARKINSON'S?

When you advocate for your person with Parkinson's, be it during a medical appointment or in a conversation with friends, it increases awareness of Parkinson's, builds community, and creates the opportunity for people to solve problems together.

Advocating for your person with Parkinson's often involves educating others about what your person experiences. Getting people to understand Parkinson's isn't easy. Stereotypes, misunderstandings, healthcare, and the media have done an excellent job of either misrepresenting or stigmatizing people with Parkinson's ever since it was first recognized as a disease. It would be exhausting to teach everyone you interact with about Parkinson's, but finding people with whom you can share your story is a step toward creating a more inclusive environment. Authentic conversations about Parkinson's can provide meaningful support.

> *Some people—sometimes even close family members—just see the person with Parkinson's who is active, who rides a bike all the time, who is healthy. They don't see the times when the person is OFF or when they're struggling."*
>
> — PAT DONAHOO

You can advocate for your person with Parkinson's in multiple ways. One particularly helpful way is to be an advocate during their medical appointments or hospital stays. We often hear from care partners that the person with Parkinson's "plays up to the physician during appointments," saying that everything is fine even when it isn't. For this reason, it is often essential for the care partner to go to appointments, record the conversation (if allowed) or take notes, and make sure the physician is listening to you and your person with Parkinson's.

Your person with Parkinson's motor symptoms can worsen when they are coping with a medical illness in addition to Parkinson's; so, during a hospital stay, they might not be able to move as well as they usually can. They might also find that some symptoms, such as tremor, dyskinesia, and freezing, worsen during a hospital stay or emergency room visit. Similarly, confusion and hallucinations can occur or worsen in the setting of medical stress or because of new medications, such as narcotics for pain, or sedatives for sleep, anxiety, or agitation. Being aware that these symptoms might appear or worsen can help you feel more prepared to advocate for your loved one and inform others about what might occur and how to treat your person's symptoms during a hospital stay.

You can find several documents on the *Every Victory Counts* **website** to help you capture and share medical information. A few to complete and take with you during your person's hospital stay include:

- 📄Prepare for Your Hospital Stay
- 📄Medical Summary for Your Physician's Appointment
- 📄Daily Medication Log
- 📄Current Symptoms Summary

These worksheets will make it easier for your person's hospital care team to understand and recognize their symptoms; they may not be familiar with problems such as dyskinesia, ON/OFF fluctuations, and freezing of gait. Be sure you let your person's hospital care team know how your person's movement and abilities change during a medication's ON and OFF times. This information will also help the hospital care team understand why it is vital that your person gets their medications on time, every time.

You can also be an advocate for your person when you're out in social settings. If you notice your person is uncomfortable with Parkinson's being the topic of conversation, step in and redirect the conversation. If you have a dinner scheduled with friends and your person is exhausted, decline the invite or reschedule. These actions remind your person that you're in their corner.

You can also be a Parkinson's advocate at local, state, and national levels, influencing funding decisions, healthcare policies, and the research needed to find a cure.

"What do I need to know about palliative care for Parkinson's? In what ways can it help?"

By Janis M. Miyasaki, MD, MEd, FRCPC, FAAN

Dr. Balfour Balmont, a surgeon in Montreal, Canada, coined the term palliative care, meaning "to relieve symptoms" for those with prostate cancer. These days, palliative care is widely used in reference to care that encompasses a holistic, team-based approach that shifts the focus of care from an individual patient to the patient and their family together. At its best, palliative care "provides relief from pain and other distressing symptoms, affirms life, and regards dying as a normal process; intends to neither hasten nor postpone death; integrates the psychological and spiritual aspects of patient care; offers a support system to help the family cope during the patient's illness and their own bereavement; uses a team-based approach; will enhance quality of life; and is applicable early in the course of illness, including when life-sustaining therapies are used."

For people living with Parkinson's, there are many moments when palliative care can be beneficial. If palliative care resources were readily available, people with Parkinson's could access them at the time of diagnosis to address existential suffering; that is, to answer questions such as, "Why has this happened to me? How can I be hopeful? How can I go forward from this diagnosis?"

WHAT IS THE DIFFERENCE BETWEEN HOSPICE AND PALLIATIVE CARE?

There is a saying: "All hospice is palliative care, but not all palliative care is hospice." In the US, *hospice* refers to care provided either in-home or in day programs for those in the last six months of life. A hospice has a medical director who is a palliative care specialist and will work with nurses, physical therapists, occupational therapists, speech-language pathologists, respiratory therapists, and others to provide supportive care in the home or in supportive living. People may remain enrolled past the six-month duration, but the expectation is that those enrolled in hospice are imminently dying.

In contrast, *palliative care* is provided throughout an illness or chronic condition. A study of palliative care for those with metastatic cancer found that those enrolled in palliative care survived longer than those who weren't; thus, it's natural for those with a complex, chronic disease, such as Parkinson's, to be referred to palliative care. Various stages have been proposed for referral, including unresolved symptoms, care partner burnout, need for coordinated care, existential suffering, and complex neuropsychiatric complications of illness, such as psychosis (hallucinations or delusions) or severe anxiety.

The first dedicated palliative care clinic for Parkinson's was established in 2007 at the University of Toronto, Canada. Using a multidisciplinary approach (including a pastoral counselor, palliative care physician, movement disorder specialist, nurse, and care coordinator), the clinic demonstrated that people with Parkinson's had a symptom burden like those with metastatic cancer and responded similarly favorably to interventions. The most improved symptoms as measured by this study were constipation, dysphagia (difficulty swallowing), anxiety, pain, and drowsiness.

WHAT SHOULD I EXPECT MY PERSON WITH PARKINSON'S TO EXPERIENCE AT A PALLIATIVE CARE CLINIC?

A well-developed palliative care program should consist of a multidisciplinary team. Depending on the clinic, your person with Parkinson's may be seen by all providers at once or by all providers rotating through the clinic room. The latter approach is more efficient for the clinic staff, even though this can result in a long day for you and can generate many individual lists of follow-up tasks.

In addition, the clinic should offer services to you and other family members since supporting families during the long journey of Parkinson's is crucial. Providing families with options to approach challenging situations is part of the team's role. The team can also affirm that your instincts are correct in dealing with a situation or gently steer you in the right direction. This can reduce the natural guilt and stress that may be associated with watching your loved one struggle with Parkinson's.

Helping people with Parkinson's and their families build a web of support in the community should be a palliative care team's role, as well. Your palliative care team should be familiar with local resources, their suitability, and cost to help you navigate this complex healthcare system. Although this may be the first time you and your family are facing this condition, the clinic faces this scenario daily, and they are well prepared to guide you. You are not alone.

If such a time comes, your person's palliative care team should also offer support and care for people who are dying. Particularly in the US, ambulatory palliative care teams coordinate with local hospices for those ready to transition to hospice care.

Palliative care for Parkinson's is expanding in North America and throughout the world. Dedicated teams recognize the burden that Parkinson's can be for people living with it and their care partners and provide holistic and practical care throughout the long journey of living with Parkinson's. Many families living with Parkinson's share that the palliative care clinic is "THE most care" they have ever received. Pursuing a referral to a palliative care team for your person with Parkinson's may be your first step in addressing the complexities associated with Parkinson's care.

About Janis M. Miyasaki

Janis Miyasaki is a graduate of the University of Toronto, where she completed medical school, residency, and a movement disorders fellowship under Dr. Anthony Lang. She joined the University of Alberta faculty of medicine and dentistry in 2014 following 22 years at the University of Toronto. In 2015, Dr. Miyasaki became the director of the movement disorders program comprising seven neurologists and a dedicated interdisciplinary team. She has held leadership positions at the University of Toronto, the University of Alberta, the International Parkinson Disease and Movement Disorder Society, and the American Academy of Neurology. Dr. Miyasaki founded the first dedicated palliative care program for Parkinson's and related disorders at the University of Toronto in 2007. Since then, she has published original research on this topic and is viewed as the founder of palliative care for Parkinson's. In 2015, Dr. Miyasaki established the Complex Neurologic Symptoms Clinic at the Kaye Edmonton Clinic, University of Alberta, with Dr. Wendy Johnston, an expert in ALS. This program provides care to all neurologic patients with palliative care needs.

WHAT DOES THE DATA SAY ABOUT THE ROLE OF A CARE PARTNER?

In 2020, a Kyowa Kirin survey of 695 Parkinson's care partners highlighted how this role comes with both significant emotional gains and emotional tolls. 78% of the care partners surveyed said the role is the most rewarding one they've ever had. Still, nearly as many said it also negatively impacts their emotional and mental health. Most said that despite feeling lonely and being overloaded with daily responsibilities, they are hesitant to ask for help, even though they need additional support. And four in five care partners agreed that they'd had a challenging time adjusting to life as a care partner.

This data makes clear that being a care partner can be both rewarding and a significant stressor. Whether you have just begun caring for someone diagnosed with Parkinson's, are dealing with a substantial progression of symptoms, or have been caring for someone who has lived with Parkinson's for a long time, the role can take its toll on you. Therefore, you must take time to learn about everyday stressors, signs of burnout, changing family dynamics, and other care partner challenges. Once you know what you might face, you can take action and feel empowered to face whatever comes your way.

"How can I live well today as a Parkinson's care partner?"

By Angela Robb

My relationship with Parkinson's began with a mouse click.

I met my husband, Karl, in an online chat room almost 25 years ago. Our first discussions were all about getting to know one another and playing 20 Questions.

Our conversations were easy, and his dry sense of humor came shining through our instant message exchanges. Within the first week or so, he told me that he was diagnosed with Parkinson's four years prior. His disclosure did not alarm me, and I remember asking, "Don't older people usually get Parkinson's?"

I married Karl, never having known him without Parkinson's. I love him, but I do not love the disease. We acknowledge that it is part of our lives, but we do not allow it to be all our lives. We decided early on in our lives together to start our own business and work from home. At the time, we were in our mid-30s, and we didn't want to postpone our desire to own our own business. Since the progression of Parkinson's is unpredictable, we decided to grab the bull by the horns and pursue our dreams.

We have adapted our goals and plans to account for the unpredictability of Parkinson's, which can change by the day or even by the moment. We do our best to plan, but we usually have a backup strategy–not just for Karl, the Parkinson's, or his medications–but for me, too. We ask ourselves questions: Do we have enough energy to tackle that task? Would we be more prepared to take on that task tomorrow with more energy or stamina? Communication, honesty, and self-awareness allow us to share how we feel and come up with a mutually agreeable approach.

That's why I've always considered myself a "care partner." Karl and I had a few discussions about our roles in this part of our life together, and we consider ourselves partners on the journey of living with Parkinson's. Others may think of themselves as "caregivers," and indeed, it's up to individuals to determine which term (or any other) best fits their personal preference and specific responsibilities.

For simplicity here, I'll use the term care partner to describe any person who has primary responsibility for assisting with the care and decision-making for a person living with Parkinson's.

Care partner is not my primary identity (although I've become somewhat knowledgeable on the subject and do my best to pass on what I've learned to others). When I meet people, it's not the first thing I tell them, but I think I would be doing myself a disservice not to acknowledge that it is one of the hats I wear. My husband says, "If you don't accept your diagnosis, fighting illness becomes even harder." I believe that the same idea holds true for care partners. Acceptance does not mean giving in to Parkinson's; it means being prepared for the road ahead and wherever it takes you.

There is some peace to be found in acknowledging this role, but it doesn't mean that I must give up another part of myself to make room. Parkinson's will not define Karl, and it's not going to define me, either. I'd like to share some of the things I've learned with you so that you can find your own peace in caring for someone living with Parkinson's.

Anyone who has cared for another knows the temptation to forego one's own needs when someone else's needs seem more pressing. For many years, as I visited with other care partners, I stressed my firm belief that we needed to take care of ourselves first so that we could care for our loved ones with Parkinson's.

It's so easy to put ourselves last on the care list. We put our children, spouses, family, home, work, pets, and more ahead of "me." When a chronic disease like Parkinson's is part of the equation, there's an even greater tendency to make our loved ones the number one priority. Yet, if we don't care for ourselves, who will?

It is vitally important that care partners have a depth of self-knowledge and are willing to ask, "How am I doing today?" or "How am I doing at this moment?" My realization of this

PART ONE: WHAT DOES IT MEAN TO BE A CARE PARTNER?

fact came from my study of Reiki and mindfulness meditation. My self-knowledge evolved, and I'm so happy that it did. I only wish that I had come to it sooner! I find myself checking in on my mental, emotional, and physical awareness. This is something that you must do by yourself, for yourself. As much as your loved one, family, or friends may ask you how you are doing, they may not be prepared for your honest answer. Most care partners will not respond truthfully anyway. The honest answer is found in being with yourself and reflecting honestly on the whole package.

I find that posing meaningful questions to myself is helpful. Once you begin an internal dialogue with yourself, you will find questions suited to you and your personal needs. Here are some examples of mine:

- How balanced do I feel mentally today?
- How do I physically feel today? Are there areas that need some attention?
- How much time can I make for myself to meditate and exercise today?
- How can I best care for myself today?

This personal reflection helps me acknowledge my own needs and gives me pause to make sure that I attend to them. It's a simple exercise, but it works. I encourage you to try it.

About Angela Robb

Angela Robb is a 25-year wife and care partner for her husband Karl, who was diagnosed with young onset Parkinson's more than 30 years ago. She and Karl co-authored the book Dealing and Healing with Parkinson's Disease and Other Health Conditions: A Workbook for Body, Mind, and Spirit. *She is a co-editor at ASoftVoice.com, a contributor and community team member at ParkinsonsDisease.net, and a Reiki Master. Angela has advocated for caregiver issues by sharing her experiences on Capitol Hill, at various regional and national Parkinson's conferences, and as a presenter at the World Parkinson Congress. In 2015, Angela was honored at The White House as a Champion of Change in Parkinson's Disease.*

Part Two: Care Partners After a Parkinson's Diagnosis

Dear husband,

After 16 years with Parkinson's, more than half our marriage, I want to thank you for standing by me. I know it hasn't been easy on you. This is a condition that affects both us and our marriage. But somehow, we have laughed and loved our way through it. We take our marriage vows seriously, and we have been through "sickness and health." However, I know we have had choices along the way. I know it's frustrating for you when I need to exercise and don't want to. I know it hurts you when I'm in pain. But isn't that what marriage is? It's the good times and the not-so-great times. It's the joy of seeing DBS work so well. But it's also the "Parkie days," the days I don't want to get out of bed, and the apathy and anxiety get to me. It is those days that I see your love. It's when you encourage me without pushing. When you bring me my meds or offer to rub my dystonic toes. It's when you say, "Let's just take a short walk." It's all the times you took care of the kids before DBS when I couldn't do anything but cry. It's sticking with me during COVID when we have only each other. It's hearing you have cancer and that the "care partner" job may someday have to switch.

We can't predict the future. After almost 30 years together, the only thing we can rely on is each other. I love you. And I know you love me. Together we will face whatever they throw at us.

Love, Jill

MY PARTNER IS NEWLY DIAGNOSED WITH YOPD. WHAT SHOULD WE TELL OUR CHILDREN?

One common care partner challenge for people with children is deciding when and how to share the news of the diagnosis. Work closely with your person with Parkinson's to understand how they feel about sharing the news. When they're ready, you can be their advocate and a resource for your children as well.

The way you and your person with Parkinson's share the diagnosis with your children will vary based on their age and maturity level. No one knows your children better than you do; so, you probably know what they can and can't handle. With children of all ages, take time to check in with them about what they're thinking and feeling. Giving them opportunities to put their concerns into words can help them make sense of their feelings and allow for a more open and honest dialogue.

Children seven and younger. If your children are seven or younger, you can give them the basic facts about Parkinson's, talk about things that might change, and stress that there are medications and actions your person can take to manage their symptoms. Be clear and consistent in what you say, and don't let the conversation go on too long. Remember, children pick up on a lot and will often mirror your demeanor. Maintaining a positive attitude allows them to go on as before.

Children eight to 14. With children ages eight to 14 (approximately), explain the diagnosis in a simple, factual way and don't overburden them with excessive scientific terms or non-motor symptoms like hallucinations that might sound scary. Remind them that their loved one with Parkinson's still loves them. Retaining as much normalcy as possible and giving them a sense of control will help them process the diagnosis. Be ready for them to ask questions, either in the moment or later, especially if they decide to research Parkinson's independently. If they do that, be sure to stress the importance of seeking reliable sources and show them how to do that.

> *I used to go with my dad to the store when he was really shaky so I could help him with the shopping cart and make change more easily. He needed extra hands, and I was happy to help him, even when I was little, like nine or ten years old."*
>
> **— KELSEY PHINNEY**

Teenagers and older. For teenagers and older children, leave the dialogue open and communicate with them as your person with Parkinson's health changes or they experience new symptoms. This helps your children know that you and your person with Parkinson's want to keep them in the loop. After learning about the diagnosis, older children will often focus on what they can do. Depending on where your person is in the process, you can either assure them that nothing much is changing or suggest some specific actions they can take to help. For example, you may suggest they can help by cooking dinner once a week or by helping to hold your loved one—or you—accountable for completing an exercise goal every day.

"How might my partner's Parkinson's diagnosis impact our family dynamics?"

By Nancy Bivins, LMSW

A Parkinson's diagnosis leaves each family member with their own set of questions, such as:

- Will my spouse be able to continue working at their job's required level of speed and accuracy?
- How will this affect our relationship as a couple?
- Will we have to give up our plans to travel?
- When will we tell our friends?
- Is Dad going to be able to go on our annual fishing trip?
- Can Grandma get down on the floor and play with us?
- And so on

After a family member is diagnosed with Parkinson's, one of the most immediate changes is the shifting of family roles and identities. Before the diagnosis, family members probably thought of themselves as the spouse, the partner, the daughter, the son, the grandchild, the sibling. Then, suddenly, their identity may also include care partner.

So, what should you keep in mind?

Rest often and ask for help when needed. Since responsibilities are shared in a family, it's reasonable to expect that when a family member living with Parkinson's can no longer do something, another person will automatically assume the task. However, it is essential to realize that some of these tasks might not be something you or other family members should take on. Sometimes, better options include hiring professional help, asking family or friends to step in, adjusting your standards (for example, mow the lawn once every other week instead of twice per week, or hire someone to do the task), or eliminating the task altogether (for example, by letting someone else host the annual summer party).

Make connecting a priority. People with many friendships are less likely to experience sadness, loneliness, low self-esteem, and problems with eating and sleeping. If your loved one is experiencing shame or embarrassment due to Parkinson's symptoms, however, they may self-isolate and begin avoiding social gatherings where you once went as a family. Because social isolation is a gradual process, it's possible to not even be aware of this change. Isolation can affect the whole family, so be proactive and encourage your family member with Parkinson's to stay connected.

PART TWO: CARE PARTNERS AFTER A PARKINSON'S DIAGNOSIS

Make nighttime adjustments. If your loved one with Parkinson's has significant nighttime needs, know that some care partners and families find success in hiring overnight help. With this arrangement, the person living with Parkinson's is safe—the in-home care professional meets their needs—and the rest of the family can rest and feel prepared to provide quality care the next day. Because this is an expensive and sometimes invasive option, it is out of reach for many families. Another recommendation is for you to sleep in a separate room, if possible, and use a monitor to check on your person remotely. You may find other solutions that work well for you, such as asking a family member or close friend to provide respite care at night once a week to give you a regular break.

Find the right support group. A support group is an excellent resource for care partners, whether the people in the group are spouses, children, or friends of people living with Parkinson's. It's easier to share your concerns with a group that is facing similar issues. Support group chemistry will vary, so be sure to visit a support group at least three times before deciding to stay or to move on. If, after your third visit, you're not convinced that it's the right group for you, try a different group—but please don't give up! Great, lasting friendships are often forged in support groups, and you and other family members may gain countless benefits from taking part.

Make the most of today and every day. Enjoy life and live it to the fullest! Although Parkinson's will affect many different aspects of your family life now, try not to make it the central aspect. I often hear people in the exercise classes at the Muhammad Ali Parkinson Center shouting with enthusiasm, "I may have Parkinson's, but Parkinson's doesn't have me!" While this may sound simplistic, it's a critical idea for people with Parkinson's and their families to take to heart.

About Nancy Bivins

Nancy Bivins received her Master of Social Work degree from Arizona State University. She serves seniors and people living with disabilities. Eight years ago, she joined the community outreach team at the Muhammad Ali Parkinson Center in Phoenix. This position has allowed her to meet people living with Parkinson's and their families and provide encouragement, support, and information as they face the challenge of living well.

SHOULD I ATTEND PHYSICIAN APPOINTMENTS WITH MY PERSON WITH PARKINSON'S?

Yes, whenever possible. Most care partners we know recommend you attend appointments to offer your own perspective, mention things you may have noticed that your person hasn't, take notes, and be an advocate for your person. You and your person with Parkinson's are both impacted significantly by Parkinson's and are familiar with its effects on your everyday lives. If the typical medical appointments focus only on the person with Parkinson's, let the Parkinson's healthcare provider know that you are an active member of the care team by contributing during the appointments. Another great tip we hear from many care partners is to record physician appointments, which you can do easily from your smartphone. This way, when you both get home, you can review what your physician said, and you have the recording in case either of you has trouble remembering the conversation.

SHOULD I BE RESPONSIBLE FOR ORGANIZING (FILL IN THE BLANK: MEDICAL APPOINTMENTS, MEDICATION LISTS, HEALTH CARE DIRECTIVES, ETC.)?

Your responsibilities in these matters will likely change as your person's Parkinson's progresses. In the early stages, your person may not need help with scheduling appointments and completing paperwork. It is best to encourage your person with Parkinson's to do as much independently as they can in those cases. However, it is often advised that you do work together during the early stages to prepare legal documents and advance directives, including a living will and medical power of attorney.

> *I always say, 'It's your decision, not mine, but here's what I think.' My role is to give input. Once she makes the decision, I try to make sure we see it through and get the outcome she's looking for."*
>
> — MIKE

WE HAVE HEARD COUNTLESS PEOPLE TALK ABOUT HOW IMPORTANT EXERCISE IS FOR PEOPLE WITH PARKINSON'S, BUT MY PERSON WITH PARKINSON'S WON'T DO IT. WHAT SHOULD I DO? HOW CAN I GET THEM TO EXERCISE?

With everything we know about the benefits of exercise for Parkinson's, it seems like getting people to exercise would be easy. But that is often far from the case. Here are just a few reasons why it might be hard to get started:

- Many people who get a diagnosis of Parkinson's do not have an active lifestyle. When they are now told they must exercise regularly, it might be too much. Education around exercise and finding exercise programs of interest are keys to success but no guarantee.

PART TWO: CARE PARTNERS AFTER A PARKINSON'S DIAGNOSIS

- Many people who get a diagnosis of Parkinson's have been dealing with pain, motor symptoms, trouble sleeping, fatigue, declining mobility, and possibly depression for many years.
- Exercise can be difficult, and it takes time to form a habit and adapt.

Here's advice from our Ambassadors—some who are people with Parkinson's, some who are care partners to people with Parkinson's, and some who work with people with Parkinson's. We hope that one of their ideas will speak to you so that you can encourage and support your person to get moving, even when they don't feel like it.

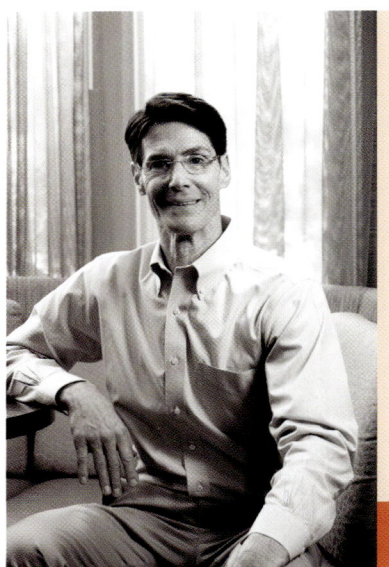

"You cannot get someone to engage in a serious wellness plan, including exercise, until they feel that there is hope. They have to trust that there's something meaningful to look forward to and live for. For people who are newly diagnosed and for anyone who is having trouble motivating themselves to exercise, I would reiterate that this is not the beginning of the end, but the beginning of a new journey that can be rewarding and happy if you allow it to be."

— STEVE HOVEY

"For me, my care partner Pat is a big help. If he doesn't ride, I probably won't go out, but I'm much happier once he gets me outside to exercise. For people who haven't been exercising, it's essential to start small with something they enjoy and gradually build up towards more intense exercise. Group classes can also help because you get the necessary exercise and, at the same time, you build a community of support and friends. I also find online resources, specifically videos, to be motivational and encouraging."

— CIDNEY DONAHOO

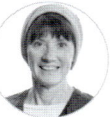

" *For anyone trying to encourage a person with Parkinson's to exercise, I would encourage them to do the following:*

- *Offer education to provide information about why exercise is so critical. Resources like the* Every Victory Counts *manual, pamphlets from Rock Steady Boxing, and scientific research can help explain the importance of exercise.*

- *Communicate with your person with Parkinson's to open an encouraging dialogue that motivates them to exercise. Sometimes a little nudging from a healthcare professional can also help to send a stronger message.*

- *The invitation makes exercise seem more accessible because a care partner who invites opportunities to move rather than nagging can be much more successful. It also allows honest dialogue about the barriers that your person with Parkinson's may feel."*

— KAT HILL

" *Since isolation is so dangerous for people with neurological diseases, including Parkinson's, I think it should be a priority to spend time with friends, and that time together can be spent exercising. I would also remind people who have difficulty getting motivated to read all the scientific evidence on how important exercise is for people with Parkinson's. Getting outside to exercise has also been shown to be beneficial because it helps with sleep by contributing to our circadian rhythms. Since sleep is a problem for people with Parkinson's, it's even more important that people get outside and exercise to counteract sleep problems."*

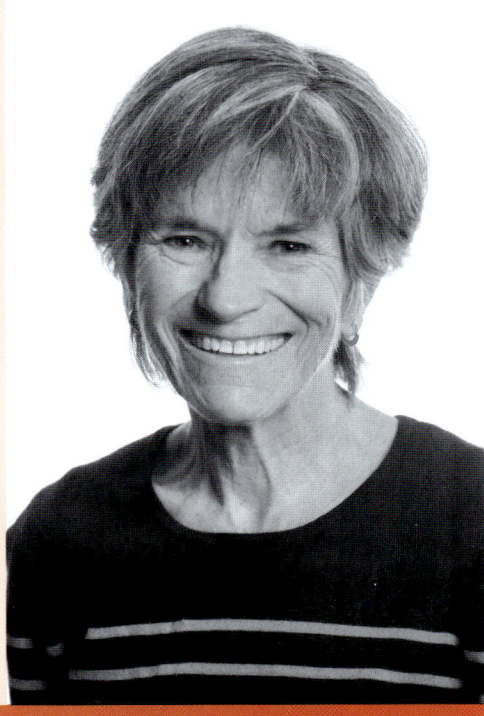

— PATTI BURNETT

PART TWO: CARE PARTNERS AFTER A PARKINSON'S DIAGNOSIS

> "Invite, encourage, support, and repeat, repeat, repeat. Recruit friends to reach out. Group classes are great, and it's always much easier to walk into something with a buddy. However, I also believe that the person with Parkinson's must want it themselves too. You have to be a fighter and be willing to try."
>
> — JULIE FITZGERALD

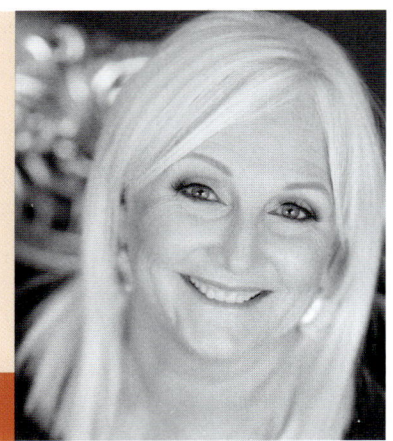

> "One of the most effective ways to combat apathy is by being part of an engaged community with people who keep each other accountable. Often it is people with Parkinson's who are the best at motivating each other, rather than care partners."
>
> — AMY CARLSON

> "One great way to get people with Parkinson's involved in exercise is to include them in exercise studies as parts of clinical trials or other Parkinson's research. I also believe that teaching behavior and attitude changes can help people go from a sedentary lifestyle to an active one. For many people, having an exercise buddy, being part of a class, or having a personal trainer can keep people accountable. I've found that people are less likely to adhere to regular exercise schedules without that outside stimulation. Success breeds success, and the more you exercise, the better you feel."
>
> — LORRAINE WILSON

> "When I work with people with Parkinson's and their care partners, I encourage a multidisciplinary approach to care to increase interest and participation. We focus on educating people with Parkinson's and their families on the importance of participation in symptom management and disease progression. It's also important to find local programs that are of interest so that the person with Parkinson's is motivated to be engaged. It truly takes a village to achieve these goals, but it's certainly possible!"
>
> — JULIA WOOD

EVERY VICTORY COUNTS

" *If I were working with someone with Parkinson's who was having difficulty getting motivated to exercise, I would contact a local Parkinson's group or a Davis Phinney Foundation Ambassador and do the following:*

- *Find Parkinson's-specific classes or classes that people in the local Parkinson's community particularly enjoy. The environment of the gym and the coaches make a difference.*

- *If your person with Parkinson's still drives, suggest they drive those to exercise classes who cannot drive. My husband does this, giving him a sense of responsibility and a feeling that he is making a difference. Once these people start boxing or spinning or whatever is their choice, they feel different, and the symptoms are at bay, at least for a little while. Over time, the exercise class becomes a support group for them, and they wouldn't miss it for the world.*

- *Even if you're having trouble motivating your person with Parkinson's to exercise, don't nag them. Just make sure they know that you are there for them and be persistent in a caring way."*

— COE LONDON

" *Getting out with friends and family is one of the most important ways to encourage exercise because it keeps you accountable and changes your attitude."*

— KEVIN SCHMID

" *Encouraging a reluctant person with Parkinson's to begin exercise is certainly a community effort, so getting the person involved in a community can help. Inviting the person to a class or event, especially those that accept Silver Sneakers cards, is a sure way to help them find the motivation to be and live well."*

— RICH WILDAU

PART TWO: CARE PARTNERS AFTER A PARKINSON'S DIAGNOSIS

> *"When I meet people with Parkinson's who need help getting started with exercise and taking control of their diagnosis, I like to offer them a variety of exercise opportunities. I think it's also important to speak to a movement disorder specialist because many of them will prescribe exercise. It can also be beneficial to attend a support group, especially because many of them will have exercise sections."*
>
> — JOE O'CONNOR

You have heard repeatedly that your attitude, your own behavior, and your consistent and compassionate presence in your person's life count a great deal. Do your best to help them find a type of exercise they enjoy but remember to get out there and take care of yourself, too.

"My person with Parkinson's is hesitant to tell friends and co-workers about their diagnosis. Why might this be?"

By Allan Cole, PhD

One of the first questions many of us have after we're diagnosed is whom we should tell. Several people I know have kept their Parkinson's diagnosis private, some for a long time. For some, there may be good reasons to keep a diagnosis private. After all, Parkinson's can come with all sorts of misperceptions, naivety, and flat-out wrong assumptions about what it will mean for a person's future. However, this silence can take a toll. You likely will have to work hard to camouflage or explain away symptoms, hiding something that has become a central part of your life.

For the first ten months after my diagnosis, I stayed silent about it. All the while, I felt disingenuous and inauthentic. It was as if I were cheating on people I care about while also being unfaithful to myself, and this became more painful than having Parkinson's. However, when I began sharing my diagnosis, I felt not only relieved but empowered to live a good life with Parkinson's. Just as importantly, being open about my condition helped me meet others living with Parkinson's. I have never regretted the decision to live openly with Parkinson's; I just wish I had begun doing so sooner.

About Allan Cole

Allan Cole was diagnosed with YOPD in 2016, at age 48. Since then, he has devoted significant time and energy to raising awareness, providing education, fundraising, and writing about his own experiences of living with Parkinson's. Allan is a professor and the academic dean in the Steve Hicks School of Social Work at The University of Texas at Austin and a Professor of Psychiatry at the Dell Medical School. A prolific writer, he's published ten books and dozens of articles on various topics related to grief, anxiety, and spirituality. He's also an avid runner who believes exercise is one of the essential keys to living well with Parkinson's.

WHAT SHOULD MY PERSON WITH PARKINSON'S AND I KNOW ABOUT DISCLOSING THEIR DIAGNOSIS AT WORK?

Workplace issues are some of the more stressful topics that people with Parkinson's confront. Your financial circumstance may be the overriding concern. However, the stress from trying to keep it a secret can build to what may seem like an untenable level. This stress, in turn, can significantly increase your person's Parkinson's symptoms, and a vicious cycle may follow. Making a plan and enlisting the help of an attorney, financial planner, or another advisor knowledgeable about work, disability insurance, and long-term financial planning can provide the peace of mind your person with Parkinson's needs to bring the stress level down.

There are pros and cons to informing an employer and colleagues about a diagnosis. In an ideal workplace situation, your person won't have to spend much energy hiding their symptoms or worrying about being found out. They may find support, camaraderie, and genuine kindness from their co-workers and might even be viewed as inspirational. Conversely, revealing a Parkinson's diagnosis can lead to a hostile environment or other undesired consequences. Your person's boss and co-workers might be inflexible and unaccommodating to their situation. They might show little or no commitment to making work a positive experience for your person with Parkinson's.

Before your person decides whether to be open at work about Parkinson's, they and you should think carefully about their job, co-workers, and the people in positions of authority in their workplace.

- Is there a history of trust, a culture of flexibility and innovation, camaraderie, and teamwork?
- What is the economic and financial situation of the company?

PART TWO: CARE PARTNERS AFTER A PARKINSON'S DIAGNOSIS

- Do your person's unique skills and experience make them irreplaceable?
- Are there protections to prevent your person from being pushed out?
- Does your person with Parkinson's have disability insurance through their workplace or independently?

These are tough questions that deserve serious consideration. Whether to be open at work is an individual decision and learning your options will help you and your person with Parkinson's in your deliberations. Know your person's rights and consult with an attorney specializing in disability, discrimination, or workplace issues. They can help you decide how much and how soon your person wants to disclose at work and understand what may be covered under disability laws.

"My person with Parkinson's isn't experiencing any burdensome motor symptoms. Should they begin taking medication anyway?"

By Aaron Haug, MD

The purpose of medications for Parkinson's is to improve quality of life. This might enable a person to work longer, complete daily activities more easily, or pick up or continue a hobby. Most movement disorder specialists, myself included, recommend treating motor symptoms—tremor, stiffness, and slowness—to the point that they're no longer interfering with quality of life.

The concern that people with Parkinson's often have is that they don't want to "use up" their medication options. This is an important point. It's a misconception that medications "only work for five years" or some other time frame. Two things are going on that contribute to this belief.

The first thing is how long a person has had Parkinson's, and the other thing is how long that person has been on medications for Parkinson's. Indeed, medications work best in the early years of living with Parkinson's, with more significant benefits and a lower likelihood of motor fluctuations and dyskinesias. However, this has as much to do with how many years a person has had Parkinson's as it does with how many years they have been on medications. When a person has lived with Parkinson's for more years, they usually need more treatment. The medicine doesn't stop working, but it's also not a cure. The progression of Parkinson's leads to more symptoms. There are multiple ways to address this, including increasing the dose of one medicine or using multiple medicines together. The guiding principle is to start medication if symptoms negatively impact quality of life and adjust medications over time to maximize quality of life.

About Aaron Haug

Aaron Haug is a neurologist and movement disorder specialist with HealthONE Neurology Specialists in Colorado. He attended undergraduate at Creighton University and then earned his medical degree at the University of Kansas. He completed a neurology residency and a fellowship in movement disorders at the University of Colorado, including a year as Chief Resident. His medical interests include Parkinson's, tremor, other movement disorders, deep brain stimulation (DBS), and botulinum toxin injections to treat neurological conditions. Outside the office, he likes spending time with his wife and kids, running, skiing, and following Colorado Rockies baseball.

HOW CAN I ENCOURAGE MY PERSON WITH PARKINSON'S TO MAINTAIN THEIR INDEPENDENCE AS SYMPTOMS START PROGRESSING?

Encourage your person with Parkinson's to manage as much as possible and adjust that load as you and they need. Determine what they *can* do before you determine what they can't do. By encouraging and expecting your person with Parkinson's to do tasks they're still capable of doing, you keep them connected to a sense of purpose and usefulness while also relieving some of your burdens and maintaining your own independence.

Every situation is unique. Your person with Parkinson's may want nothing more than to keep doing everything independently, or they may feel so defeated by their diagnosis or progression that they don't want to do anything. Both can present challenges. As a care partner, it's essential to learn the balance between helping and enabling and between encouraging and dismissing. Maintaining constant communication can help you know which path is best at any given moment.

MAINTAIN YOUR OWN INDEPENDENCE AND IDENTITY

Being a Parkinson's care partner can be equally demanding and rewarding, but no matter your circumstances, there will likely be times when you feel you are losing yourself in the role. A few data points from the 2020 care partner survey conducted by Kyowa Kirin illustrate this well:

- Parkinson's care partners spend an average of 45 hours per week caring for someone with Parkinson's, with their top responsibilities being emotional support (92%), managing medical appointments (81%), transportation to and from appointments (81%), and helping with memory issues (74%).

PART TWO: CARE PARTNERS AFTER A PARKINSON'S DIAGNOSIS

- While 86% of Parkinson's care partners agree that the role makes them feel very lonely sometimes, four out of five feel guilty when asking for help from others or taking breaks from being a care partner (81%).
- Nearly one in three (30%) agree that finding time to balance their personal or social life is a big challenge they typically face as a care partner.

The key to being an effective care partner is prioritizing self-care, feeling supported by your person with Parkinson's, and having something to call your own.

> *I don't compartmentalize wife and care partner, but I know it's important to take time for myself. I play tennis a couple of times a week, babysit, and enjoy the grandkids."*
>
> — NANCY HOVEY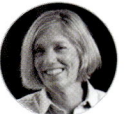

Fortunately, there are several strategies you can use to maintain your independence while still giving your person with Parkinson's the quality care they need. Here are some strategies that might help:

- **Take self-care seriously.** Self-care is one of the most important aspects of living well. If you feel stressed or overwhelmed, try to incorporate some of these regularly:
  - Engage regularly in a hobby or activity you enjoy
  - Check in with your support system
  - Take care of yourself: exercise, eat healthy food, and drink water to restore your energy
  - Practice mindfulness, meditation, or another calming activity
  - Communicate with your loved one about how you're feeling
  - Let your emotions out. Talk to a therapist/counselor or good friend
  - Be kind to yourself and practice self-compassion
  - Practice gratitude every day
- **Acknowledge your limits.** Find out what is possible for you to achieve and stick to it, but don't push your boundaries. As we explained earlier, that is a great way to encounter care partner burnout. Know when and where to ask for help.
- **Make a list of duties you can delegate.** Then delegate. While you might be hesitant to ask other people to do things you typically take care of, you'll likely be a more effective care partner if you take some responsibilities off your plate. Remember that people want to help but likely need direction. Ask them to drop off a meal, take a walk with your person with Parkinson's, or pick up your dry cleaning or some groceries.

EVERY VICTORY COUNTS

- **Establish and maintain consistent routines.** Parkinson's is continually changing, but having consistent routines can make unexpected moments and unplanned detours easier to manage.

- **Make sure your care team is well-rounded.** The more help your person with Parkinson's has, the more help you will have. Invite friends, family members, physicians, therapists, social workers, support groups, spiritual leaders/clergy members, or volunteers into your life to help you maintain balance and get the care you need.

- **Have fun!** Don't forget to set aside time to do things you enjoy with your person with Parkinson's. For some, fun may include travel or planning big adventures. For others, it may involve reading books over coffee or hunkering down to watch TV. Whatever it is you like to do together, keep doing that.

Remember, most people will live a very long time with Parkinson's; so, it's important to stay connected to what you want and what's important to you while you're on this path. Parkinson's is part of your life, but it is not your whole life, just as it is not your loved one's whole life. Take steps every day to be your own person, find joy, and care for yourself just as you care for your person with Parkinson's.

MY PERSON WITH PARKINSON'S IS MY PARENT AND LIVES IN ANOTHER STATE. HOW CAN I HELP? WHAT CAN I DO TO STAY INVOLVED? WHAT'S MY ROLE? WHAT SHOULD I NOT DO?

Even if you are not the primary care partner for your person with Parkinson's or the person on their care team closest to them, you can still play an instrumental role in supporting them. A good first step is to ask your parent's primary care partner what they need. You could help with respite care, or you could be helpful by working with the insurance company over an unresolved issue. Be prepared to do what is asked and encourage the primary care partner to delegate tasks and share the workload.

Every person with Parkinson's experiences it differently, so take time to understand how your parent is impacted by it physically, emotionally, and mentally. Then, help them based on your skillset and what they need. If your parent's primary care partner is someone other than you, ask that person how you can help them as well. You can be a great relief and resource for your parent's primary care partner.

Keep in mind that just as it may not be easy for you to shift into the role of a care partner, it may not be easy for a parent to receive care from their child. The shifting dynamic from one where the parent made all the decisions to one where the adult child is driving decision-making requires time and trust to work through. Ask your parent(s) what kind of role they would like you to take and how you can be most helpful but be assertive and let them know tactfully what you observe and what you think they need. From a distance, you may observe changes that those closest to the person with Parkinson's may have missed.

Educate yourself on the constellation of Parkinson's symptoms to better interpret what is going on. Parkinson's comes with good days and bad; you will not always be able to tell what kind of day your parent is having by their outward appearance or behavior or by how they sound during a phone or video call. Just because your person with Parkinson's may not display any signs of feeling bad, it does not mean they aren't experiencing symptoms. They might be "playing up" for you, or they may be good at hiding their symptoms. Invite your parent to share how they're feeling by saying things like, "I'd love to know more about how you're feeling if you're up for talking about it." This kind of invitation shows that you can't understand all they are feeling but that you want to.

> *For a child who doesn't live with their parent who has Parkinson's, they worry a lot. 'Will he be okay? Is he going to fall?' The key is preparation. The better the person with Parkinson's is prepared, the better the care partner will feel."*
> — **NANCY HOVEY**

"What is it like to grow up with a parent who has Parkinson's?"

By Matthew Ater

Parkinson's is hard. Having a parent with Parkinson's is hard. But as easy as it sometimes is to think, "Woe is me; this is too hard," it's not too hard.

Here's how I know:

My mom has Parkinson's. And her mom and sister have Parkinson's. In other words, it's a true family "gift." Looking back, though, although Parkinson's runs in our family, it doesn't define my family or me.

When I was seven, my mom was diagnosed with young onset Parkinson's. My younger brother was four. Now that I'm twenty-three, I honestly can't remember much about my mom before her diagnosis. I do remember, however, that her Parkinson's didn't just "happen overnight" and that it took its sweet time to develop. Specifically, I remember her hand starting to cramp and one side getting off-kilter. Still, like every kid, I was focused on my world. I wanted to ride my bike and play with my friends. And I did, all while noticing that my mom was very thoughtful with her Parkinson's. She didn't try to hide it from my brother or me. As far back as I can remember, it was talked about in our family just like we talked about the weather. I was just another kid who did what other kids did, except at times, I also had to help my mom in and out of the car, take her hand when she struggled with balance, and move more slowly around a store. Other than that, nothing was different about my childhood because my mom had Parkinson's.

Parkinson's doesn't hit you like a train, and boom, your life is over. Parkinson's is an aspect of life that fills in the cracks. When I think about how Parkinson's has changed our lives, I believe the change has been more positive than negative. As weird as it is to say that a progressive neurological condition is good, I stand by that belief. When I was a kid, Parkinson's was why we could skip the lines at Disney World and park in the handicapped spots at the mall when it was crowded. But as I grew up and matured, Parkinson's became the thing that motivated me to go to the gym with my mom so that I could help her work out—and, surprise, it helped me stay in shape at the same time.

Most importantly, though, more than the fun of skipping lines at Disney, it is the intangible benefits that have proven to be the most valuable. I know that Parkinson's has made me more patient and kinder, more empathetic, and more motivated. It has also taught me to slow down, to focus, and to look for good things in life when everything seems difficult.

Before my mom had deep brain stimulation (DBS), my parents worked a lot. My brother and I would fight, and our mom and dad would get upset. Normal family stuff. That changed a lot after my mom's brain surgery. We slowed down. We realized that happiness can be a choice we make and that our family was the most important thing in the world. My parents retired earlier than they had planned because DBS gave them their lives back, and as a result, we moved to California. All those plans and dreams I used to hear my mom and dad talk about started to happen. Yes, my mom was slower, and she couldn't walk as far, and she showed up to my lacrosse games with a cane, but she was ALWAYS there.

I watched as my mom became very involved in the Parkinson's community. She started working with others, sharing her story with others living with young onset Parkinson's, and helping in the community however she could. And she made dang sure that my brother and I helped as well.

Parkinson's is hard; it truly is. There are bad days when we cry and feel broken down by it. On those days, it is tough. On the days that seem exceptionally difficult, I've learned those days are that way because we let them be. The days when we are smiling and happy and the world is full of light are the days when we get to decide what we want them to be. I've learned to slow down and appreciate the good things in life. Just because Parkinson's is in the picture, why stop living? Besides, I've learned that life is better at a little slower pace anyway. When you slow down, you see more, hear more, feel more, and have more of yourself to give to others.

PART TWO: CARE PARTNERS AFTER A PARKINSON'S DIAGNOSIS

I overheard my mom a couple of years ago talking to a woman newly diagnosed with Parkinson's. The woman was in tears. She thought her life was over and that Parkinson's was a death sentence. My mom told her this: "Have a pity party. Be sad. Be angry. Life is hard, and it's not fair. You are allowed to have your pity party. But you aren't allowed to give up. So have your pity party and then get back up and get on the horse and go."

That stuck with me. Parkinson's is hard. Life is hard. But not too hard. Be upset, be mad, be sad, but don't give up. Parkinson's doesn't take away your life. It just makes you slow down and enjoy the ride a little differently.

About Matthew Ater

Matthew Ater is a recent college graduate living in Chester, England. He has a strong personal connection to Parkinson's; his mother, grandmother, and aunt have lived with Parkinson's for most of his life. Matthew has been involved with the Parkinson's community for many years through his mother's work and enjoys sharing his story with new care partners. Matthew prides himself on helping others in any way he can and has found the Parkinson's community to be a space where he can assist others while being part of a strong network of people who truly understand one another.

MY PERSON WITH PARKINSON'S LIVES ALONE. HOW CAN I HELP?

One meaningful way you can help is by ensuring your person's home environment sets them up for safe, productive, and enjoyable living. In part three of this manual, we'll share some ways you can help create a safe space, and for many more home safety tips, check out our 🏠 Home Safety Checklist in this manual's appendix.

The best thing to do is ask them what they need. A direct ask is almost always more helpful than an open-ended question. For example, ask, "Would it be helpful if I came over and helped with your laundry and some housework tomorrow?" instead of saying, "Let me know if I can help or if there's anything I can do for you." Although it seems like a nice idea to make an open-ended offer, it puts more work on the person living with Parkinson's. If you make a direct ask, it is easier for them to assess whether your offer would be helpful and give you a yes or no. Making things easier for them is a true gift.

Other gifts you can give—perhaps the most valuable ones—are your time and attention. Outside of taking medication, people living with Parkinson's benefit most from two things: exercise and connection. Give them both by asking your loved one to take a walk (if you do this outside, you also give them a third benefit—sunshine!). Call them every Sunday afternoon to catch up. Take them lunch. Practice yoga together one morning a week. Stop by to chat a few times a month. Whatever you do, stay connected.

MY PERSON WITH PARKINSON'S IS MY SPOUSE. SINCE THEIR PARKINSON'S DIAGNOSIS, WE HAVE NOT BEEN ON THE SAME PAGE IN OUR DESIRE FOR INTIMACY. WILL THIS CHANGE? WHAT SHOULD WE DO?

Just as aging affects a couple's sex life, so does Parkinson's. For a care partner who is in an intimate relationship with a person with Parkinson's, the emotional impact of the diagnosis can interfere with the desire for sexual intimacy. So too can sexual dysfunction, a common Parkinson's non-motor symptom. Because many people living with Parkinson's and their partners are reluctant to bring up this issue, it often goes unmentioned and untreated. The good news is that through open communication, counseling, and (if needed) adjustments to your person's medication regimen, you and your person with Parkinson's can maintain a healthy and enjoyable sex life.

At the time of diagnosis, you and your person with Parkinson's may be too distracted to initiate sex or participate with any interest. Discussing emotions and intimacy isn't always easy, so know that it may take time to adjust and adapt to the idea of living with Parkinson's and everything it entails.

On the other hand, some people with Parkinson's report concerns about hypersexuality and compulsive sexual behavior. In people with Parkinson's, this behavior, also referred to as an impulse control disorder (ICD), is often a side effect of dopaminergic therapy. Read on for more information about ICDs and talk with your person's physician immediately if they experience these symptoms since they can often be treated by diminishing the dose of dopamine agonists.

Parkinson's motor symptoms, including tremor, stiffness, rigidity, and dyskinesia, can all interfere with sexual activity. So too can non-motor symptoms such as fatigue, excessive salivation, sweating, anxiety, apathy, depression, and cognitive changes. And while some Parkinson's medications, such as dopamine agonists, can increase sexual interest and activity, others, such as certain antidepressants, can do just the opposite.

The most common sexual problem for men living with Parkinson's is erectile dysfunction (ED). ED often goes together with depression, so for some people, taking an antidepressant can help. Some antidepressants, however, can decrease sex drive and cause ED; so, work closely with your Parkinson's care team to discuss medications that are less likely to contribute to ED. Other ED treatments include different medications, physical and/or talk therapy, and surgical implants.

PART TWO: CARE PARTNERS AFTER A PARKINSON'S DIAGNOSIS

Women living with Parkinson's typically report that a loss of lubrication and involuntary urination during sex are their biggest concerns. Because many women with Parkinson's experience decreased lubrication, sexual activity can be painful. Other symptoms women report include decreased sex drive and problems with orgasm. As with men who experience ED, women who feel concerned by a loss of sexual desire or other issues can work with their physicians to see if medication changes help. Other treatment options include adding lubrication, timing sex for ON periods when symptoms are well controlled, and working with a sex counselor or other therapist for personalized strategies.

You may find the topic of sexual dysfunction gets little to no priority during medical visits, even though it may be high on your or your loved one's list. If these concerns aren't getting enough attention, ask your physician to refer you to the professional best suited to address them. Counseling, especially with a licensed sexologist, can help couples overcome many of the sexual intimacy barriers they experience.

As we mentioned, aging naturally leads to changes in needs and desires, and Parkinson's will likely lead to these changes as well. Remember, though, that intimacy means many things. Physical touch, such as holding your partner's hand or hugging them, is an expression of intimacy. Refining and redefining what intimacy means to you can be a meaningful and freeing conversation between you and your partner.

MY PERSON WITH PARKINSON'S IS EXPERIENCING COMPULSIVE BEHAVIORS. WHAT IS HAPPENING?

Impulse control disorders (ICDs), including compulsive gambling, sexual behaviors, shopping, and eating, are common in people with Parkinson's who also take dopamine agonists (DAs), drugs sometimes used to treat the symptoms of Parkinson's. Because ICDs are not only common but can also have a profound effect on quality of life, it's important to learn about them and how they may affect your loved one with Parkinson's.

According to *Psychiatric Times*, impulse control disorders are characterized by:

- The perpetuation of repeated negative behaviors regardless of negative consequences
- Progressive lack of control over engaging in these behaviors
- Mounting tension or craving to perform these negative behaviors before acting on them
- A sense of relief or pleasure in performing these problematic behaviors

People who experience impulse control disorders may or may not plan the acts; however, the acts themselves nearly always fulfill their immediate wishes, even if they are ultimately distressing to the person and make them feel out of control.

The most common ICDs reported in people with Parkinson's are pathological gambling, hypersexuality, compulsive shopping, and compulsive eating. More than 25% of the people with ICDs have two or more of these behavioral addictions.

DOPAMINE AGONISTS

Dopamine agonists mimic the effect of dopamine in the brain. They stimulate dopamine receptors directly without being metabolized to another compound, as in the case with levodopa. Dopamine agonists are typically the most common medication used to treat Parkinson's, aside from carbidopa/levodopa, in the early stages of Parkinson's. This is because when compared to levodopa, long-term use of dopamine agonists may be less likely to lead to motor complications and, if they do develop, they may be less severe. In later stages of Parkinson's, carbidopa/levodopa and dopamine agonists are often taken in conjunction.

One of the benefits of dopamine agonists is that compared with levodopa, they have a longer half-life—they stay active in the body longer—and can have a more immediate effect on motor symptoms, especially if the immediate release option is taken.

Some of the most common side effects of dopamine agonists are nausea, low blood pressure, leg swelling, drowsiness, sudden "sleep attacks," and hallucinations. And in the most severe cases, impulse control disorders can be a side effect of dopamine agonists due to the receptors in the brain that dopamine agonists impact the most.

WHAT MAKES SOMEONE MORE SUSCEPTIBLE TO DEVELOPING ICDS?

Other than taking dopamine agonists, there are a variety of factors that put someone at a higher risk of developing impulse control disorders, such as:

- Being male
- Age at time of diagnosis (YOPD)
- Longer duration of living with Parkinson's
- History of drug abuse
- History of gambling addiction
- Impulsive sensation personality traits
- Family history of psychiatric disorders
- Depression
- Overuse of dopaminergic medications due to dopamine dysregulation syndrome (DDS)

HOW DO IMPULSE CONTROL DISORDERS IMPACT PEOPLE WITH PARKINSON'S AND THEIR CARE PARTNERS?

ICDs can reduce the quality of life for the person with Parkinson's and their care partner. In some of the more severe cases, ICDs cause financial ruin, divorce, loss of employment, and increased health risks.

ICDs can cause people to feel shameful, embarrassed, and weak. They may lie to hide their addictions, act in secrecy, and withdraw from family members for fear of being found out.

In some instances, people who have developed an ICD must also reconcile that they get some level of satisfaction and pleasure from their addiction, even though it could be wreaking havoc on their lives and their most important relationships. Fortunately, being knowledgeable about ICDs, risk factors, and causes is an essential step for minimizing the impact on daily life.

WHAT'S THE TREATMENT FOR IMPULSE CONTROL DISORDERS?

The most important thing to remember about impulse control disorders in people with Parkinson's is that it's a medical condition, not the result of personal weakness. If help is sought, it is possible to get better.

All ICD behaviors are on a continuum, and where they fall on that continuum and how destructive the ICD is to a person's life will indicate the kind of treatment needed. For example, a male who begins taking dopamine agonists may become much more sexual than he had been in the past. He may want sex all the time with his partner, which only seems like a big deal because this is a new desire. However, that doesn't necessarily mean his desire for more sex is destructive. In this case, he may need counseling more than he needs medical treatment. If his sexual behaviors become pathological and destructive, that's when a medical approach would be advised.

When the behaviors are severe and destructive, the first line of treatment is to reduce the last medication that was changed in treating Parkinson's symptoms. In most cases having to do with pathological gambling, reducing or discontinuing the dopamine agonist reduced or eliminated the severity of the ICD.

People with compulsive gambling, spending, or eating typically respond well to dopamine agonist reduction. In contrast, people with punding (a compulsive need to carry out a repetitive motor behavior) benefit from reducing levodopa. The population with problems resulting from hyper-hedonistic behaviors—excessive and insatiable actions that increase pleasure—may benefit from reducing either the dopamine agonist or levodopa.

Some people experience withdrawal symptoms when they stop taking their dopamine agonist; a severe condition called dopamine agonist withdrawal syndrome (DAWS). According to Melissa J. Nirenberg from the Department of Neurology at the NYU School of

Medicine, DAWS is "a severe, stereotyped cluster of physical and psychological symptoms that correlate with dopamine agonist withdrawal in a dose-dependent manner, cause clinically significant distress or social/occupational dysfunction, are refractory to levodopa and other dopaminergic medications, and cannot be accounted for by other clinical factors."

DAWS can be very challenging to manage. In this case, physicians will often put the person back on the dopamine agonist and then very slowly titrate them off. This process can take a long time and controlling the ICD in the meantime can be a significant challenge. The ongoing challenge for physicians is that reducing the dose of a dopamine agonist or eliminating it can cause distressing symptoms for the person with Parkinson's, such as decreased motor control or an increase in non-motor symptoms.

Like many addictions, the therapies designed to curb or eliminate ICDs seek to replace the previously spent time engaging in destructive behavior. Therefore, it's critical to help your person find something else to fill that time. Part of doing that is finding a support system or being the support system while your person with Parkinson's is looking for something new to focus on during vulnerable times.

WHAT CAN I DO IF MY PERSON WITH PARKINSON'S DEVELOPS AN IMPULSE CONTROL DISORDER?

The best treatment for ICDs is prevention. And as a care partner, you are in a great position to advocate early and often for your person with Parkinson's. Fortunately, physicians are much more judicious than they used to be when prescribing dopamine agonists. However, it's still important to be one step ahead of the drugs if your person with Parkinson's and their physicians decide that a dopamine agonist is the best course of treatment.

Here are a few things you can do:

- Request a detailed counseling or information session before beginning dopamine agonist therapy. (One of our community members told us how frustrated she was that her husband's physician never talked to them about the potential severity of dopamine agonist side effects. ICDs occur in enough cases with people who take dopamine agonists that physicians should be more forthcoming about them. As a care partner, you can advocate for that information now that you know more about them.)

- Do not be afraid to question your person with Parkinson's about unexplained absences, secretive behavior, irritability, hiding evidence of ICDs, and monetary consequences. Be sure to share this information with their physicians.

- Normalize their behaviors and remind them it's a result of Parkinson's and medications and not their fault. Normalizing what's happening may make them more inclined to share their concerns with you.

PART TWO: CARE PARTNERS AFTER A PARKINSON'S DIAGNOSIS

- Be on the lookout for increased insomnia, missing meals, missing doses of medication, financial issues, and absences from work, as these can all be potential red flags for the presence of ICDs.

- If the ICD is on a continuum that together you decide is manageable, work with your person with Parkinson's to develop a plan and strategies for managing the ICD. The more included your person is, the more likely they will follow through on the interventions. You want to give them as much freedom and autonomy as you can so they can still be in control of their own life, without letting go of so much that they are a danger to themselves or others.

Impulse control disorders can be highly stressful and cause a lot of pain for you and your person with Parkinson's. But it is possible to get help and treatment to reduce or eliminate their presence.

WHAT'S NEXT?

If your loved one is experiencing impulse control disorders, reach out right away and work closely with their physician, ideally their movement disorder specialist, to assess their situation and create a treatment plan that's right for them. No two people experience ICDs in the same way; so, it's critical to understand and evaluate all potential options. Throughout the process, be sure to note how your person feels, how they behave, and how medications or therapies impact them so their physicians can keep an up-to-date record of their experience.

> Dearest Bill,
>
> You have been my partner in so many ways during our 41-year marriage and before that, too. Those dating days of discovering the person you are and being drawn to your generous spirit. From cultivating the flower gardens together to bringing two beautiful sons into the world, we have stood by one another with the promise never to abandon the other in difficult times.
>
> Now we face what may be the defining partnership of our lives....
> WE have Parkinson's.
>
> You suffer my highs and lows, my speedy and not-so-speedy times, my shakes, and my freezes.
>
> But through them all, I know that you stand at my side, never judging me or wishing to escape our covenant. Trusting your dedication to me gives me the strength and courage to continue to try, work, pray, laugh, and forge forward.
>
> »

Not only are you my partner and cheerleader, but my inventor, too. How many times have you built or made something that was strictly to make my life easier? There were lifts for the furniture, multiple ramps and thresholds, and the knee block under the piano.

I recognize that my diagnosis has changed your life, and yet you hold no bitterness towards me. You have affirmed our commitment to one another over and over, especially when Parkinson's made me weak and insecure. Your loving caress and gift of music always brought me back to the present, living one day, one moment, at a time.

Times ahead will be more than challenging, and they will require your patience. To laugh away the stress of it all, let's vow to spend a few minutes every day remembering some particularly happy time/event. Then let's dream up something we want to do together before one of us is gone. We have so much to be thankful for and yet to enjoy if we can only have the right frame of mind. With God's help, we will get to the end of life with no regrets and happy hearts.

With love and eternal gratitude, Jan

MY PERSON WITH PARKINSON'S HAS MORE FREQUENT OFF PERIODS THAN THEY DID A FEW YEARS AGO. HOW CAN I HELP?

The 2020 Kyowa Kirin care partner survey showed that while nine out of ten Parkinson's care partners are optimistic about Parkinson's treatments, just as many feel that managing medication, gauging when it stops working, and knowing how to help with pharmacological treatments can be significant challenges.

Everyone with Parkinson's responds to medications differently, and your person's routine is unique to them. However, knowing that carbidopa/levodopa is the gold-standard treatment for Parkinson's, we want to offer advice about how to help your loved one get the most out of it if it's part of their medication regimen.

(For more about Parkinson's medications—the most current, in-depth lists of drug names, side effects, contraindications, and additional information—be sure to head to the medication page of our *Every Victory Counts* website.)

Levodopa and ON times. Levodopa acts to help with slowness, stiffness, and tremor and can be used in conjunction with other medications to address the same symptoms. Carbidopa is almost always combined with levodopa to enable more levodopa to reach the brain. It is also added to control nausea, which is a side effect of levodopa.

Although the terms ON and OFF have been used to describe responses to levodopa therapy for more than 50 years, there is still no universally agreed-upon definition for the term OFF. OFF periods occur when a person's Parkinson's medication isn't working optimally, and their motor and non-motor symptoms return. OFF is much more nuanced than this, but understanding its scientific causes can help you help your person with Parkinson's minimize it in their daily life.

> *I know it's important that I don't get wrapped up in myself. When Cidney is experiencing OFF times and symptoms she needs help with, I try to stay calm and relaxed, so I can help her with what she needs right then."*
>
> — PAT DONAHOO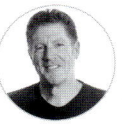

Levodopa—a central nervous system agent—helps minimize symptoms because it is converted to dopamine in the brain. OFF times take place when levodopa is no longer working well enough to suppress Parkinson's symptoms. What, though, causes levodopa to stop working optimally, and what can you do to help your loved one with Parkinson's get the most from their medicine? Here, we explore some of the science behind OFF and strategies that will help maximize ON times so your loved one can live their best life with Parkinson's.

Water and ON times. To make its way from the mouth to the brain, levodopa must travel from a person's stomach to their small intestine, where it is absorbed by an extensive neutral amino acid active carrier system. A similar transport system transfers levodopa across the blood-brain barrier to the brain, where it is metabolized to produce dopamine. The more quickly levodopa reaches the small intestine, the faster it passes through the intestinal walls and the brain's carrier system. The quicker it converts to dopamine, the more quickly your person with Parkinson's will feel ON.

Movement disorder specialist Cherian Karunapuzha, MD, says the key to minimizing delayed and partial ON times is to take levodopa on an empty stomach with a full glass of water. The water "flushes" the medicine quickly to the small intestine, and the absence of food in the stomach means nothing can slow its emptying. (Tip: crushing or chewing carbidopa/levodopa or drinking it with sparkling water can also help speed the process.) Ideally, your person with Parkinson's would take each dose of levodopa one hour before a meal (to give it time to move from the stomach to the small intestine) or two hours after (the amount of time it takes for food to empty the stomach). Because this is not always possible, especially as a person's Parkinson's progresses and they take levodopa more often, encourage your loved one to take each dose at least 30 minutes before or 30 minutes after a meal—and, again, always with a tall glass of water.

Protein and ON times. The system that transports levodopa from the small intestine to the brain is the same system that transports amino acids. Both levodopa and amino acids must enter the bloodstream through the intestinal wall and then cross the blood-brain barrier to enter the brain. If too many amino acids are present along with levodopa, the medicine must "compete" with the amino acids for absorption, and it won't enter the carrier system quickly. Similarly, some amino acids compete with levodopa for absorption in the brain. Their presence when levodopa makes its way to the blood-brain barrier will delay the time it takes for the brain to transform the medication to dopamine and, therefore, decrease or delay the medication's efficacy. This, too, can lead to delayed or only partial ON times.

In the stomach, protein is broken down into amino acids, which then travel to the small intestine. For a person's levodopa to work most effectively, it should enter their small intestine when few amino acids are present; this gives it easy access to the carrier system and fewer obstacles to crossing the blood-brain barrier. To maximize ON times, your person with Parkinson's should try to avoid eating protein close to when they take their levodopa.

Constipation and ON times. Constipation can also play a significant role in levodopa absorption and ON/OFF fluctuations. In the digestive system, food makes its way from the mouth to the large intestine through the alimentary canal (esophagus, stomach, and small and large intestines). When a person's intestines aren't being emptied regularly, the levodopa they take won't make its way through the digestive system as it should, and it cannot control the person's symptoms effectively. Help your person with Parkinson's explore lifestyle and dietary changes that will minimize constipation. Having regular bowel movements means their levodopa will work most effectively, and they will experience less OFF time. (For an in-depth look at how to manage constipation, a very common non-motor symptom of Parkinson's, be sure to check out Chapter 6 of the *Every Victory Counts* **manual** or on our *Every Victory Counts* **website**.)

> *OFF times can be challenging to control, but we focus on controlling what we can. One way to be supportive is to understand what your person with Parkinson's needs from you at the moment. Whatever I can do to help him feel better, I will do. Often that means encouraging him to just sit down, relax, and regroup. Taking a rest can really help."*
>
> — NANCY HOVEY

Parkinson's progression and ON/OFF fluctuations. Although the half-life of levodopa is short (one to one-and-a-half hours), in the first stages of Parkinson's, there is sufficient synthesis and storage of dopamine in the brain's striatal neurons to keep Parkinson's symptoms at a minimum despite few doses of levodopa. However, as Parkinson's progresses, the brain produces even less dopamine. This means it must rely entirely on levodopa

PART TWO: CARE PARTNERS AFTER A PARKINSON'S DIAGNOSIS

to control Parkinson's symptoms. Yet as Parkinson's progresses, many people begin to experience fewer benefits from their medications, and the benefits may also be less consistent. This can increase wearing OFF periods and ON/OFF fluctuations.

As a care partner, you should talk with your person's physicians about how their Parkinson's—including the frequency and severity of OFF times—has changed over time. In addition to dietary modifications, various adjustments can be made to their medication regimen to limit ON/OFF fluctuations and extend ON times. For some people, deep brain stimulation (DBS) or other surgical therapies can be effective ways to reduce OFF times as Parkinson's progresses. Ask your person's physicians what options might work for your person.

THE LAST TIME WE SAW A MOVEMENT DISORDER SPECIALIST, THEY SUGGESTED WE HAVE CONVERSATIONS ABOUT THINGS LIKE LIVING WILLS, ADVANCE DIRECTIVES, ETC. THAT SEEMS SO SCARY AND NOT NECESSARY RIGHT NOW. WHY WOULD THEY SUGGEST THAT?

None of us is excited about preparing for the day when we can't make decisions or are facing the end of our lives. However, planning for the future is important for everyone, not just people living with Parkinson's and their loved ones. And, when you make these kinds of plans early, you won't feel extra stress or worry about preparing at the last minute. Here, we'll look at some of the paperwork you will want to complete.

(Disclaimer: This information is meant purely for educational purposes. Nothing in this manual is offered as legal advice, and it should not be treated as such. You must not rely on the information in this manual or our companion website as an alternative to legal advice from your attorney or another professional legal service provider. If you have questions about a legal matter, consult your attorney or other professional legal services provider.)

Advance directives. According to CaringInfo.org, advance directives are "legal documents that allow you to plan and make your own end-of-life wishes known if you are unable to communicate. Advance directives consist of (1) a living will and (2) a medical (healthcare) power of attorney. A living will describes your wishes regarding medical care. With a medical power of attorney, you can appoint a person to make healthcare decisions for you in case you are unable to speak for yourself."

Living will. A living will is a legal document that specifies the types of treatments you do or do not want at the end of your life if you are ill and won't likely recover or are in a coma and are not likely to come out. As you complete your living will, you should clarify your desires related to:

- Cardiopulmonary resuscitation (CPR)
- Do not resuscitate order (DNR)
- Do not intubate order (DNI)

- Blood transfusions
- Dialysis
- Artificial nutrition and hydration
- Organ donation

Once you and your witness or witnesses sign your living will, it is legally binding. However, it goes into effect only once you are deemed incompetent AND incapacitated by at least one physician. If you are just incapacitated and are likely to get better, your living will won't go into effect.

*Be sure to revisit and revise your living will as necessary. It's good practice to review it every five years or after significant life changes to make sure it still represents your wishes.

Medical power of attorney. This should be someone you trust completely to help carry out your wishes. This is not an easy role to be in, especially if, for example, you have a large family of people who love you. When the tough decisions must be made, your medical power of attorney will have to do so even if it's not the decision everyone else in the room wants. Be careful in choosing this person and make sure they are comfortable in this role.

*Be sure to revisit this as often as necessary. Your relationships with people may change over the years, and the person you choose today may not be the same one you want in this role five years from now. In addition, the person you assign as your medical power of attorney today may die or be too ill themselves to make decisions for you in the future. Whenever this relationship changes, be sure to assign a new person you trust as soon as possible.

You must have someone who is over 18 and is not your medical power of attorney witness and countersign your documents to make them legal. Check the laws in your state, as some require a notary and others do not.

Once you've completed your documents, share them with the key people in your life, leave a copy in your home that's easy to find, and put a copy in your travel bags and leave it there so it's available if anything happens.

Advance directives are not the most exciting things to think about; however, if you care about the end of your life and the people who are likely to experience that with you, it's necessary to have them in place. And as many people who have done so remarked, having this in place gives them peace of mind, and when you're living with Parkinson's or caring for someone who is, that can be worth a great deal.

> Dear Dan,
>
> I am sure that if there were a care partner competition, you would win the gold.
>
> From the day we received my Parkinson's diagnosis, you have been nothing but supportive and encouraging. You have never let me give up hope that together we will somehow get through this, in the same way that we have met other challenges in our lives together.
>
> I could not ask for a more loving husband and partner - now for 37 years. Who knew that when we vowed to remain faithful in sickness and in health, that would include Parkinson's?
>
> Please know that if the day comes when I yell at you or do not fully appreciate all the sacrifices you have made for me, that it's most likely Parkinson's acting, not me. I pray that day never comes, but if it does, I have no doubt that you will forgive me.
>
> I love you, Patti

IS THERE ANYTHING I SHOULD THINK ABOUT WITH RESPECT TO OUR LIVING ARRANGEMENTS NOW? WHEN'S THE RIGHT TIME TO MAKE THESE DECISIONS?

In Chapter 15 of the *Every Victory Counts* **manual**, you can find an article by licensed clinical social worker Jessica Shurer that describes planning for long-term care and the many types of care facilities that are available. There is also an article by Bud Rockhill with advice about home care and home healthcare. Both Jessica and Bud recommend thinking about all of this before a crisis happens that might necessitate a rushed move to a care facility. Be sure to check out their advice in terms of how to plan ahead. Here, we share more about what to think about now, before your person's Parkinson's progresses to later stages.

The most important thing to consider is the safety of your person's home environment. Here are some general home safety guidelines for people living with Parkinson's.

- Decrease clutter. Place furniture so that your person with Parkinson's has wide walkways and can move around easily. Decreasing clutter in their physical space not only reduces tripping hazards but also helps to reduce mental clutter and distractions, allowing for greater focus and calm.
- Install lever handle doorknobs instead of circular knobs for easier opening.

- Install grab bars throughout your person's home. (Seek advice from an occupational therapist on proper placement first.)

- Ensure chairs in the house are stable (not on wheels), have armrests, and are the adequate seat height to make standing up and sitting down easier.

- Be sure a communication system is in place and easily accessible in every room and hallway that your person uses. This could be a video surveillance system, phone, alarm button, or medical alert necklace or bracelet. (This is especially important for people in the later stages of Parkinson's, but it's good to be thinking about now.)

- Give two or three trusted individuals keys to your person's home in case your loved one needs them to come by to help. Compile their contact information and share it with each person on the care team if they're comfortable with that. Or use a lockbox and key, garage door remote code, or a smart lock so you can offer these trusted people easy access to your person's home in case of an emergency.

- Consider a doorbell that offers a camera view so your person can see who is at the door from afar.

- Consider getting a natural gas detector for your person's home. This can be lifesaving, especially if your person has a diminished sense of smell due to Parkinson's.

- Consider in-home exercise equipment for exercise solutions in lousy weather.

- Request a visit from a physical therapist and/or occupational therapist who knows the ins and out of Parkinson's to address your person's needs and offer solutions.

- Organize the kitchen so that frequently used foods, cookware, and utensils are within easy reach.

For many more home safety tips, check out our **Home Safety Checklist** in this manual's appendix.

Have you begun thinking about whether it makes sense to downsize? For some families, downsizing allows them to not only create the safest space possible for the person with Parkinson's (by choosing a smaller one-story home or a condo, for example), but it allows them to save money they can put toward various aspects of care down the road. It takes time to downsize out of a home you may have lived in for decades; start the process early.

HOW CAN I MAKE SURE PARKINSON'S DOESN'T BECOME THE CENTER OF EVERY CONVERSATION?

Although Parkinson's is part of your life, it's essential to spend time together and with friends when Parkinson's isn't the most important person in the room. Take time to connect with your person in ways that you did pre-Parkinson's. Did you spend Friday evenings at dinner parties with friends? Were Wednesday mornings set aside for your shared runs or yoga practice? Did you have daily routines like watching a game show together, taking a walk after dinner, or enjoying coffee together first thing in the morning? Think about the everyday activities that brought you joy before the Parkinson's diagnosis, and make sure you're still taking time to do them together while talking about something other than Parkinson's.

Of course, some of these activities will change. Not everything will continue the way it did before Parkinson's was a part of your lives. Adapt, stay flexible, make new traditions, accept limitations, but remember that Parkinson's is a part of your lives, not your whole lives. Focusing on the big picture will help you take care of yourself, your person with Parkinson's, and your relationship together.

It is often easier to designate a Parkinson's-free zone in your home than in social settings or large gatherings. With the best of intentions, many friends and acquaintances may spend quite a bit of time asking your loved one how they're feeling and encouraging them to talk about their life with Parkinson's. Although these questions show they care, you can step in and turn the conversation away from Parkinson's by asking friends about their own lives, their families, current events, and community news. By shifting the topic to something other than Parkinson's, you can keep it from being the center of attention.

"My person with Parkinson's has been experiencing depression and/or anxiety for the past ten years, long before their Parkinson's diagnosis. How can I help them manage this symptom?"

By Roseanne D. Dobkin, PhD

If you believe your person with Parkinson's is experiencing depression and/or anxiety, talk to them about your observations and concerns. Emphasize that their symptoms are common in Parkinson's and that effective treatments for depression and anxiety are available. If you can, attend the next neurology appointment with your loved one and raise your concerns with the physician and other appropriate medical professionals. This will start a meaningful conversation and put mood changes on the physician's radar to continue to monitor.

Cognitive-behavioral therapy (also known as CBT) is one type of treatment that addresses behaviors and thought patterns that contribute to depression and anxiety. CBT is time-limited and skills-based and may be used alone or in combination with medication. It may be a handy option for people living with Parkinson's who can't tolerate (i.e., had uncomfortable side effects), do not wish to take, or have not been sufficiently helped by antidepressant or anti-anxiety medication. You can use several different CBT strategies to help people living with Parkinson's cope more effectively with symptoms of depression and anxiety and the daily stress of living with Parkinson's. CBT is also very open to care partner involvement in the therapeutic process. You may participate in treatment sessions and/or attend separate educational sessions to arm yourself with tools needed to support your loved one in their daily practice of newly acquired coping skills. Care partner involvement in treatment is encouraged, as it has been shown to further bolster depression outcomes in Parkinson's.

About Roseanne Dobkin

Roseanne Dobkin is an associate professor of psychiatry at Rutgers-Robert Wood Johnson Medical School in Piscataway, NJ. She is also a licensed psychologist in New Jersey and Delaware. Dr. Dobkin received her PhD in clinical psychology from the Medical College of Pennsylvania-Hahnemann University in Philadelphia, PA. The overarching goal of her research program is to help people with Parkinson's and their family members cope as effectively as possible with various challenges to enhance overall physical and emotional health and quality of life. To date, her research has been funded by the National Institutes of Health, the Patterson Trust Awards Program in Clinical Research, the Michael J. Fox Foundation for Parkinson's Research, the Parkinson's Unity Walk, the Parkinson's Disease Foundation (PAIR Leadership Award), and the Health Services and Research Development Division (HSR&D) of the Veteran Affairs Administration.

HOW DO I BALANCE MY WORK AND MY ROLE AS A CARE PARTNER?

As we explained earlier in this manual, maintaining your own identity is essential for living well as a Parkinson's care partner. And, for many people, a big part of their identity is connected to their career.

In the early stages of your person's Parkinson's, you may not need to make any changes to your work routine. Depending on your employer's policies, you may be able to use sick time to accompany your person to medical appointments, and there may be few other reasons you need to adjust your work schedule. You may also be able to take advantage of the Family Medical Leave Act (FMLA). This provision allows for 12 weeks of unpaid leave for medical-related purposes. Because the time off can be used on an intermittent basis, even hourly, it can provide a flexible option for days when you need to stay home to care for your person with Parkinson's or when longer time off may be required.

One important thing to remember as you learn to balance your work and your role as a care partner is that maintaining your own identity is key. A loved one's Parkinson's diagnosis does not mean the end of your career, passions, and dreams. Use the advice throughout

PART TWO: CARE PARTNERS AFTER A PARKINSON'S DIAGNOSIS

this manual to learn how to encourage your person with Parkinson's to do all they can for themselves, whom to ask for help when you need it, and what professionals can help both you and your person with Parkinson's when balancing your career and your care partner responsibilities becomes too much to manage.

WHEN IS IT TIME FOR MY PERSON WITH PARKINSON'S TO STOP DRIVING?

Driving is a complex task. It requires physical strength, mobility, good reflexes and reaction time, depth perception, good eyesight and hearing, and the ability to multi-task and keep track of many visual and spatial inputs at once. Some of the symptoms of Parkinson's can make executing all those tasks a challenge. A few symptoms that are the most troublesome when it comes to driving include:

- Tremor in legs, arms, and hands
- Decline in vision and spatial processing
- Fatigue
- Compromised balance
- Freezing that can make it difficult to get moving again after having been still
- Slower reaction time and diminished reflexes
- Decreased spatial awareness
- Side effects from taking medications such as sleepiness, blurred vision, and confusion
- Mild to severe cognitive impairment
- Decreased executive function
- Dementia

Many of the medications your person with Parkinson's may be taking can dramatically mitigate their symptoms; however, it's important that they and you remain vigilant when considering how safe they're able to be on the road. Some of the warning signs that indicate you may need to schedule a driving safety assessment for your person with Parkinson's include:

- They drive considerably slower than the rest of traffic
- They have trouble switching lanes
- They stop or slow down for no apparent reason
- They drift in and out of their lane
- They forget to use their traffic signals
- They get lost on familiar roads and routes and forget where they're going
- They experience severe bouts of fatigue or have sleep attacks

- They seem unaware of cyclists, pedestrians, and others who are sharing the road
- They are getting tickets for various infractions
- They get into fender benders, or almost get into them, often

If your person has done any of the above, it's crucial that you share your concerns with your person's physician and that you learn more about how your state handles drivers with disabilities. In some states, physicians are required to report patients who have specific medical conditions to their state Department of Motor Vehicles (DMV). Other states require physicians to report "unsafe" drivers to their state DMV, though states define "unsafe" in varied ways. Regardless of where you live, however, your person's physician should be able to refer your loved one to a Certified Driver Rehabilitation Specialist (CDRS®) if they have concerns about your person's abilities to drive safely or if you make this request for referral.

Once your loved one has completed a driving assessment, the CDRS will send their report to your loved one's physician, and it will be linked to your person's DMV profile. The CDRS's recommendations then become connected to a license. These recommendations must be measurable. For example, some of the restrictions that could be placed on a driver include:

- Can drive in daylight only
- Can drive only within a certain radius of their home
- Can drive below certain speeds only

In some states, the report gets sent to the medical board. Contact the DMV in your state to learn more about how it's done where you live.

Remember throughout the process not to minimize how big a transition like this can be for your person with Parkinson's. Many people experience anxiety and loss when their driving windows are limited or removed. If this is something your person with Parkinson's experiences, encourage them to reach out to friends or the people in their support group to share their experiences. Opening up to others who have gone through similar life transitions can be a great way to move through many of the changes that come with living with Parkinson's. You can also teach your person how to use rideshare services like Lyft or Uber or senior rideshare opportunities. Give them space to share how they feel about the possible loss of driving abilities and support them in this transition.

PART TWO: CARE PARTNERS AFTER A PARKINSON'S DIAGNOSIS

Part Three: Managing the Complications of Parkinson's

While many people in our community wish there were distinct stages of Parkinson's that everyone goes through to anticipate what's next, Parkinson's doesn't necessarily work that way. Some people experience more severe symptoms than others, but not on typical timelines. So, in this section, we address complications like hallucinations, cognitive decline, and big dips in quality of life due to increased symptoms.

Dear Leisa,

This letter is long overdue in writing, and I want you to know how much I have appreciated the love, care, and support you have given me over the years, especially since being diagnosed with Parkinson's. I know you carry a heavy burden and excess worry that you certainly don't deserve, and you have extra work to do to keep up with things.

I appreciate the support you have given me in my cycling adventures. Having you there to cheer us on has always been one of my favorite things. I will never forget when I got my first real road bike after being diagnosed, and it was close to our 25th anniversary. Because the bike was a silver bike, I said it was perfect because it was the anniversary color. We spent the money and bought the most expensive bike I had ever bought in my life. Since then, as I have acquired more bikes, you have handled it in stride, which I have appreciated so much.

I want you to know how grateful I am to have you as my wife and care partner.

You are the rock of our family, and I would be lost without you.

I love you!
Carl

WHAT KIND OF ACTIVITIES CAN I EXPECT TO DO AS MY PERSON'S PARKINSON'S PROGRESSES?

In addition to continuing the roles you played early on in their Parkinson's, you may now take on new responsibilities, such as:

- Scheduling and speaking up more vocally during medical appointments
- Managing outsourced and respite care
- Adapting or modifying a home to be safe and accessible
- Making end-of life-plans
- Being the executor of wills and trusts

It's always important that you speak up and offer your insights and observations during your person's medical appointments, and as your person's Parkinson's progresses, it becomes even more crucial. (Remember to get your person with Parkinson's to name you as a designated representative on a HIPAA Authorization, so you have full access to your person's medical records and updates.) You and your person with Parkinson's are impacted significantly by Parkinson's and are familiar with its effects on your everyday lives. If your typical medical appointments focus only on the person with Parkinson's, let the Parkinson's healthcare provider know that you are an active member of the care team by contributing during the appointments. On our Worksheets and Resources page of the *Every Victory Counts* **website**, we have several checklists and worksheets to help you get the most out of every medical appointment.

MY PERSON WITH PARKINSON'S IS SO WORRIED ABOUT FALLING THAT THEY DON'T WANT TO LEAVE THE HOUSE. HOW CAN I MOTIVATE THEM TO STAY CONNECTED TO OUR COMMUNITY?

There are several ways you can help. The first is to help address the root of the concern, which is falling. We take a close look at balance and how to prevent falls in Chapter 4 of the *Every Victory Counts* **manual**, and here, we share highlights for how your person can practice their balance and which professionals can help.

HOW PARKINSON'S AFFECTS BALANCE

Balance is a state of equilibrium. When you can control your body's center of mass over its base of support, you remain upright and steady. To achieve greater balance, your brain must combine information from all levels of your nervous and musculoskeletal systems. The basal ganglia, part of the brain responsible for motor control, plays a vital role in balance. The basal ganglia are also the part of the brain impacted by Parkinson's. The neurodegeneration of the SNpc dopaminergic neurons and loss of dopamine depresses the nigrostriatal pathway, and motor activity, including balance, can become impaired.

Parkinson's impact on the brain can also cause delays in a person's reaction time, speed of movements, and postural "righting reflexes." This means if your body sways off its base of support, it might take too long to "right" itself. Additionally, some of the rigidity and dyskinesia associated with Parkinson's can diminish muscular control, which increases instability. Other factors, including lightheadedness, slowness, and fatigue, can also increase the risk of falling.

HOW TO HELP YOUR PERSON WITH BALANCE CONCERNS

The good news is that although balance is one of the most vulnerable mechanisms we have, it is also one of the most re-trainable. With practice, your person with Parkinson's can improve their postural stability and even regain some of their automatic balance reflexes.

An important person to add to your person's care team, if they are not already included, is a Parkinson's physical therapist. They can assess your person's balance and work with them to develop a personalized training program to address their balance deficits. Parkinson's physical therapist Hannah Fugle says the most effective balance exercises are:

- High intensity
- Challenging and cognitively engaging (requiring your sustained attention to perform it well)
- Repetitious (taking place every day or most days of the week)
- Progressive (demanding more work and attention as your skills improve)
- Meaningful (improving your quality of life)
- Enjoyable

Help your person discover exercises that fulfill these needs. Explore with your person exercises that focus on flexibility, strength, and agility, which are key ingredients to improving balance and coordination. Activities that incorporate balance elements, such as yoga, tai chi, Pilates, the Feldenkrais Method®, boxing, and dance, are ideal for people with Parkinson's because they relieve stress and help build balance control.

HOW TO MOTIVATE YOUR PERSON TO STAY SOCIALLY CONNECTED

The second part of this care partner challenge is encouraging your person with Parkinson's to stay connected to their community. Social isolation can exacerbate your person's symptoms, put them at risk for developing other health problems, increase their chances of experiencing depression, accelerate cognitive decline, and decrease their quality of life. So, what can you do to help your person avoid the temptation to isolate and get reconnected to the world around them?

#1. Start small. Plan an outing where you can be present with your person the entire time, one that will not take much time, but that can help your person build confidence in being out in the community.

PART THREE: MANAGING THE COMPLICATIONS OF PARKINSON'S

#2. Make a deal. Talk with your person about the importance of social connections and make plans to take one action a week or to do one new activity each month with others.

#3. Explore Parkinson's-related exercise classes. Numerous exercise classes are designed specifically for people with Parkinson's and can help your person stay connected and improve their balance. Whether it's Dance for PD®, Rock Steady Boxing, Pedaling For Parkinson's, PWR4Life®, Silver Sneakers, or one of the many other activities available, these classes can be life-changing for people with Parkinson's.

"How can I make sure our home is safe for my person with advanced Parkinson's?"

By Amanda Craig, OTR/L, CBIS

So much of our lives are spent in our homes. We eat, sleep, and cultivate passions there. We create art, food, and music there. We study and educate ourselves there. And, of course, we visit others and maintain relationships there. So, home needs to be a place that supports our goals and allows us to thrive.

To help ensure your home is safe for your person with Parkinson's, an occupational therapist (OT) can visit your residence and learn about how you and your person live on a day-to-day basis. They may take measurements and ask your person with Parkinson's to perform some of their daily, typical tasks, like getting around in the bathroom, preparing food in the kitchen, getting in and out of the closet, and feeding any pets. Afterward, they will provide you and your person with Parkinson's with recommendations and potential resources that might be specific to your person's needs or general accessibility recommendations. The OT should also let you know what home changes are essential to make right away.

Depending on your person with Parkinson's needs, goals, symptoms, and lifestyle, an OT may recommend modifications to your seating arrangements and furniture, kitchen organization, lighting, bathrooms, and stairs and walkways. Additions and improvements to your home such as grab bars, push-pull doorknobs, bed canes, touch-on lights and faucets, doorbell cameras, and improved lighting can make your home not only more comfortable but safer for your loved one as well.

About Amanda Craig

Amanda Craig is a licensed occupational therapist and owner of Ada Therapy Services, PLLC in Boise, ID. Amanda provides individualized outpatient treatment for adults and adolescents experiencing functional "real life" deficits caused by neurological and chronic conditions. The therapists at Ada Therapy Services subscribe to the founding principle of occupational therapy: all people need to be active and occupied to be satisfied. Amanda completed her graduate degree in occupational therapy from Idaho State University and a bachelor's degree in business from Philadelphia University/Thomas Jefferson University in her home state of Pennsylvania.

MY PERSON WITH PARKINSON'S WAS DIAGNOSED AT AGE 48 AND IS NOW 73. THEY GREW UP AN AVID ATHLETE AND EXERCISED REGULARLY WITH PARKINSON'S UNTIL TWO YEARS AGO WHEN THEY LOST THE MOTIVATION TO CONTINUE DOING SO. THEIR PARKINSON'S HAS PROGRESSED RAPIDLY IN THE PAST FEW YEARS. HOW CAN I HELP THEM GET BACK ON TRACK?

An excellent place to start is with your person's physician, ideally their movement disorder specialist, to see if your person's medications need to be adjusted. If medication can be optimized, your person will hopefully feel better and have more motivation to get moving.

Next, if possible, seek out a Parkinson's physical therapist. As we've highlighted several times, a Parkinson's PT can work one-on-one with your person to develop a personalized fitness plan that will keep them safe while they return to regular exercise.

Another strategy is to encourage your person with Parkinson's to get a buddy and exercise together. You can also try walking while listening to music, which many people with Parkinson's say helps them with stride, gait, and balance. Start small, encouraging your person with Parkinson's to walk down your driveway and back with you while getting your mail. Join a Parkinson's exercise class as a pair, where you can both build social connections as well as fitness levels. Research physical activities that neither of you has done before and that are appropriate for your person's abilities and symptoms and learn how to do them together. Enter a fundraising event where you can earn money for a cause you support by exercising.

Focus on positive reinforcement. If your person has been a lifelong athlete, there's a good chance that once they've been reintroduced to the many benefits of moving their body, they will notice that it creates a positive cycle and improves their quality of life. If it doesn't, discuss with their physician what therapies and other treatments might help.

MY PERSON WITH PARKINSON'S HAS BECOME APATHETIC ABOUT EVERYTHING. WHAT CAN/SHOULD I DO?

Apathy means that a person lacks motivation, desire, and interest to do something. Though the cause of apathy is unclear, research indicates that it's due to a chemical imbalance and structural changes in the brain. Often apathy is more frustrating for you than your person with Parkinson's because your person has lost the capacity to care about whatever it is you are hoping they will do.

One day a care partner brought her husband to see psychiatrist Gregory Pontone, MD, MHS, because she was worried that her husband just sat on the couch all day and did nothing. Dr. Pontone asked her person with Parkinson's, "Do you know the difference between apathy and depression?" He replied, "I don't care." This is a perfect example of apathy.

Another patient of Dr. Pontone's was a lifelong baseball fan. One day when he was watching the seventh game of the world series, the power went out. When it came back on, the screen showed only snow. An hour went by, and he continued to watch the snow on the screen rather than the seventh game of the World Series. Again, he was not frustrated, upset, or depressed. He was apathetic and just didn't care.

That attitude might be acceptable for your person with Parkinson's, but it will likely cause severe frustration for you. So, it's critical to work with your person's physician to obtain an accurate diagnosis of apathy. Apathy seems to parallel cognitive decline with disorganization and memory loss, and medications for cognitive problems appear to work best for apathetic people.

In addition to experimenting with medications, if that works for your person's situation, Dr. Pontone suggests making a plan for your person to get out of the house daily. If you plan the day of activities ahead of time, your person can just step into it. Explore new places. Go for a picnic in a park you've never visited. Try out new restaurants. Connect with people in your community who haven't always been part of your social "circle." Wander around a museum that's new to you and your loved one. New and novel experiences that shake up your routine may help shake off some of the apathy your person is experiencing.

If neither medications nor setting daily schedules puts a dent in your person's apathy, ask your person's neurologist or movement disorder specialist for a referral to a specialist in this field.

HOW CAN I BE MOST HELPFUL DURING MEDICAL APPOINTMENTS?

The first action you can take is before the appointment even begins. Ahead of time, make a list of goals for the appointment, your person's most bothersome symptoms, and any new or concerning issues. Keep a diary of your person's medication schedule and use it to track symptoms, and be as detailed as possible with times, dose, etc. On the *Every Victory Counts* website, you can find several checklists and assessments that can help.

During the appointment, speak up so your person's physician can be given the full story of current symptoms. You may have noticed new symptoms or changes in symptoms that your person with Parkinson's hasn't, so being present during appointments and sharing this information is extremely helpful. It can also be helpful to record the conversation and, when you get home, discuss what the physician said. You may be surprised by how much your recollections of the appointment differ.

MY PERSON WITH PARKINSON'S IS SHOWING SIGNS OF COGNITIVE DISTRESS. WHAT SHOULD I DO?

Cognition is a general term used to describe our mental ability to process information and apply knowledge. Not only can Parkinson's slow down movement (bradykinesia), but it can also slow down one's ability to think and process information (bradyphrenia). Because Parkinson's alters many regions of the brain and the dopamine system, it can affect executive function, language, speech, comprehension, and memory. Approximately 50% of people with Parkinson's will experience cognitive changes to varying degrees.

In mild cognitive impairment, which is estimated to occur in 20-50% of people with Parkinson's, a person may still be able to work and complete day-to-day tasks, just at a slower pace or slightly reduced volume. Many people with Parkinson's can think and analyze, communicate, remember information, and function normally.

Cognitive and mood-related symptoms typically require more hands-on care than some of the mobility challenges of Parkinson's. A significant cognitive concern for many people living with Parkinson's is dementia. Most recent figures suggest that up to one-third of people living with Parkinson's will develop dementia, a significant cognitive change that affects how they live their daily lives. It can also impact a person's ability to live independently. If this is the case, the introduction of a caregiver is often necessary, even if your person's motor symptoms are still being well managed.

In Chapter 6 of our *Every Victory Counts* manual, we take a close look at cognitive changes and what your person can do to stay cognitively strong. You can explore that chapter or our information about cognition online, but in the meantime, we want to share a message from Mark Mapstone, PhD, about how changes in cognition relate to you as a care partner.

PART THREE: MANAGING THE COMPLICATIONS OF PARKINSON'S

"How can I respond in a helpful way when I notice my person with Parkinson's is experiencing cognitive problems?"

By Mark Mapstone, PhD

Patience and understanding are key. Cognitive changes may be challenging to comprehend or accept, and as a result, people living with Parkinson's may minimize or deny cognitive changes. In some cases, they may not be able to recognize that these changes are happening. In this situation, repeatedly pointing out and trying to convince your loved one of their cognitive lapses is rarely fruitful. The goal is to be supportive and understanding and help with tasks to decrease frustration and, if necessary, to ensure safety. Have frank discussions about any cognitive changes with your loved one's Parkinson's physician. For specific cognitive tasks, patience and understanding can go a long way. It may be tempting to finish sentences for someone struggling with word-finding but be patient. Allow several seconds before jumping in. That mental search strengthens brain networks, and it may make it easier to come up with the word next time.

It's essential to be aware that cognitive changes can be confusing, frustrating, and just as disruptive as motor changes. We all need to understand that people with Parkinson's are giving their best with what they have, and what they have is different now.

About Mark Mapstone

Mark Mapstone is professor of neurology at the University of California, Irvine School of Medicine, where he is also a member of the Institute for Memory Impairments and Neurological Disorders (IMIND). He holds an adjunct appointment at the University of Rochester. His research focuses on early detection of neurological disease, especially Alzheimer's and Parkinson's, using cognitive tests and biomarkers obtained from blood. He has a special interest in developing strategies to maintain successful cognitive aging. In the clinic, he specializes in cognitive assessment of older adults with suspected brain disease.

Dr. Mapstone earned a PhD in clinical psychology at Northwestern University and completed fellowship training in neuropsychology and experimental therapeutics at the University of Rochester.

He has authored more than 100 manuscripts and abstracts and is the recipient of a Career Development Award from the National Institute on Aging. His research has been funded by the National Institutes of Health, the Michael J. Fox Foundation, and the Department of Defense.

"I have heard that as Parkinson's progresses, a person can develop Parkinson's psychosis. What does this look like?"

By Cherian Karunapuzha, MD

Psychosis is a non-motor symptom of Parkinson's. Parkinson's psychosis manifests in different ways, such as hallucinations–seeing, hearing, or feeling something that is not there; and delusions–irrational beliefs or convictions. People living with Parkinson's have a 50% risk of developing psychosis at some point, and it can occur at all stages of Parkinson's. In the later stages of Parkinson's, psychosis can be an integral feature of Parkinson's dementia. When psychosis occurs earlier in Parkinson's, it usually coincides with starting certain medication classes or when pushing to higher doses. However, it can also occur without any provoking factors in the middle stages of the disease.

The term psychosis encompasses several features, including a false sense of presence, illusions, hallucinations, and delusions. A false sense of presence is the feeling that someone is standing beside you or is in the room with you, but when you turn around, no one is there. An illusion is a distortion or misinterpretation of something real that was sensed, like mistaking a belt for a snake. On the other hand, a hallucination is an imaginary sensation perceived without anything in the environment to provoke it. It's like seeing an imaginary dog in the corner of your room when there is nothing there. A delusion is a false, irrational belief which cannot be shaken despite being given evidence to the contrary.

The first step toward addressing Parkinson's psychosis is to understand and accept that this is a common non-motor symptom of Parkinson's and to report these symptoms early so your wellness team can keep track of them over time and offer treatment strategies. The earlier psychotic symptoms are noticed and addressed with your person's care team, the better you can manage them to give your person the best possible quality of life.

About Cherian Karunapuzha

Cherian Karunapuzha is a movement disorder specialist, assistant professor of neurology at the University of Oklahoma Health Sciences Center, and director of the OU Parkinson's Disease & Movement Disorders Center. He completed his internship in internal medicine, residency in adult neurology, and a fellowship in movement disorders at the University of Texas Southwestern Medical Center, Dallas. He is a member of the AAN and holds board certification from the American Board of Psychiatry and Neurology.

Dr. Karunapuzha is a keen clinical educator who has received several teaching awards and is a frequently invited speaker for CME programs. Focused on community medicine, he has developed clinics for the uninsured in tandem with the patient support groups so as to improve statewide access to movement disorder specialists as well as access to research studies.

I'VE NOTICED THAT MY PERSON WITH PARKINSON'S SEEMS TO BE HALLUCINATING, BUT WHEN I MENTION IT, THEY DENY IT. WHAT SHOULD I DO?

If the person you care for experiences a hallucination, there are a few things you'll want to do in the moment and others you'll want to do when the moment passes.

The most important thing to remember is to resist the temptation to talk your person out of their hallucination. They are actively experiencing it, and by trying to talk them out of it, they may either feel like they aren't being heard or that their experience is being diminished.

What matters in that moment are their safety and your reassurance that they're going to be okay. You might calmly say, "I understand that you're seeing X. I'm not having that experience, and I just want you to know that everything is going to be okay. There's nothing dangerous happening here, and you're safe."

Other strategies Joanne Hamilton, PhD, ABPP-CN of Advanced Neurobehavioral Health of Southern California, shared with us are to:

- Turn on all the lights to make the room as bright as possible, as hallucinations often happen in low lights
- Have the person look closely at what they see to help reset the brain and make the hallucination end

- If the person does not have insight (meaning they are having a hallucination but are not aware they're having it), give them a lot of reassurance, provide a distraction, move into a different room, or suggest a new activity

Here are a few actions you can take once the hallucination has passed:

- Talk to the person about it (most of the time, even if the person does not have insight, they will remember it when it's over)
- Tell their physician and offer as much detail about the episode you can remember, such as time of day, location, and anything else that may be relevant, like how tired or hungry/full they were
- Be sure to keep light switches in convenient locations. Since waking up and going to bed are the most prevalent times for people with Parkinson's to hallucinate, turn lights on fast, and make sure they're bright
- Eliminate or reduce shadows in the house, and be careful of where you place mirrors and reflective surfaces, as they can play games with the mind
- Investigate any environmental triggers that could be causing hallucinations with more frequency or regularity

MY PERSON WITH PARKINSON'S HALLUCINATES FREQUENTLY BUT ISN'T BOTHERED BY THEM. IS IT OKAY TO LET IT GO?

We discussed this topic with Christopher Goetz, MD, professor of neurological sciences and pharmacology at Rush University Medical Center in Chicago. Here's what he had to say: "There's a long history of a sort of humorous approach to these hallucinations. Some physicians call them 'benign hallucinations.' But they are not benign because Parkinson's is progressive. I've done a study where I treated people with Parkinson's who had these minor hallucinations with either medication or strategies to keep the hallucinations quiet because I don't want these hallucinations to progress. The data showed that the people I treated at a low level had a better outcome than those who received no treatment for their hallucinations. We have to acknowledge that Parkinson's is a progressive condition. Calling something a 'benign hallucination' connotes that we don't have to worry about it. I think we do have to worry about it. And we now have treatments."

Even if your person isn't bothered by their hallucinations, it's important that you discuss them with a specialist to get personalized advice for how to manage the symptom. For more advice about communicating about hallucinations with a physician, check out our webinar recording with Dr. Goetz on the *Every Victory Counts* **website**.

MY PERSON WITH PARKINSON'S IS HAVING VERY EXTREME HALLUCINATIONS, AND I'M SCARED WHEN THEY HAPPEN. I DON'T KNOW HOW TO CALM THEM DOWN. WHAT CAN I DO WHEN IT'S HAPPENING?

Here's what you can do in the moment:

- Stay as calm and patient as you can
- Remove any objects in the room that could pose a danger to your person with Parkinson's, yourself, or anyone else
- Clear space so there are no tripping hazards, and your person can move around freely
- Reassure your person that everything is going to be okay
- If the person becomes aggressive, minimize your movements and remain calm
- Ask the person to talk to you about what they are feeling and really listen, so they don't feel threatened
- If you feel like you or they are in danger, call 911

Here are a few actions you can take once the hallucination has passed:

- Inform your person's physician immediately
- Educate others who may care for the person how to handle the situation if it happens when they are with your person
- If your person is open to it, discuss the occurrence with them and ask them to explain what the experience is like for them and if there's anything different you could do next time
- Seek expert advice if you feel like you need support in managing these episodes

IN THE PAST YEAR, MY PERSON WITH PARKINSON'S HAS BEGUN EXPERIENCING DELUSIONS AND FREQUENTLY ACCUSES ME OF HAVING AN AFFAIR. NO AMOUNT OF DENIAL CAN CONVINCE THEM OTHERWISE. WHAT CAN I DO?

Delusions are specific and fixed beliefs that are very real and true to the person experiencing them. They can contradict all semblance of reality and rational thought, but no amount of convincing could change what the person believes is true. Additionally, if you try to convince someone experiencing a delusion that it's not true, they can become suspicious and doubt you, making an already difficult situation even worse.

Delusions happen much less frequently than hallucinations. Only about 10% of people with Parkinson's experience them, but because they're often ongoing, involuntary, and feel very real to the person, they can be much more difficult to manage and treat.

The most common delusions people with Parkinson's experience are:
- The belief that their spouse is being unfaithful
- The belief that their care partner is poisoning them with their medications
- The belief that people are stealing their stuff, or they're going to steal it

The single most important thing to do if your person is experiencing delusions is to tell their physician right away. The earlier they know what's going on, the sooner they can begin interventions to help your person feel better. Once you share your concerns, your person's physician will typically do a clinical evaluation, review your person's medications and dosage, assess their lifestyle, and determine the severity of the symptoms. Depending on what they find, they may refer your person to counseling or therapy, adjust their medication, change their medication, eliminate a particular medication, or do all the above. If none of those strategies work, they may try antipsychotic drug therapy to see if they can adjust chemical levels in the brain. This can bring an entirely different set of problems with it, so it's important to be invested every step along the way and be sure you're well-informed before you move in that direction.

If the person you're caring for experiences confusion or delusions, here's what you can do in the moment:
- Stay as calm and patient as you can and remember that this belief has nothing to do with you and only with what is going on in their mind
- Remove any objects in the room that could pose a danger to them or anyone else
- Clear space so there are no tripping hazards and so it's easy for the person to move around
- Do not try to reason with the person or convince them why their belief is false
- Reassure them that everything is going to be okay
- If the person becomes aggressive, minimize your movements and remain calm
- Ask the person to talk to you about what they are feeling and really listen to them, so they don't feel threatened
- If you feel like you or they are in danger, call 911

Here are a few actions you can take once the delusion has passed:
- Inform your person's physician immediately
- Educate others who may care for your person how to handle the situation if it happens when they're around

PART THREE: MANAGING THE COMPLICATIONS OF PARKINSON'S

- If your person is open to it, discuss the episode with them and ask them to explain what the experience is like for them and if there's anything different you could do next time
- Seek expert advice if you feel like you need support in managing these episodes

HOW CAN I MANAGE THE EMOTIONAL TOLL I'M FEELING FROM MY PERSON'S PARKINSON'S DISEASE PSYCHOSIS?

Often the most challenging part of Parkinson's disease psychosis is the fear of the unknown. As a care partner, you may worry that you won't be able to help your person with Parkinson's feel safe if something does happen. The good news is you now have information on what Parkinson's disease psychosis is, the risk factors to look out for, biological and environmental triggers that can bring them on, and how to manage them if they show up.

But what about the emotional toll these types of symptoms put on you over the long term? Here are some actions you can take:

- Join a Parkinson's care partner support group if you don't already belong to one. Talk about your experiences and ask for help if you need it
- Allow others to help you care for your loved one with Parkinson's. Take breaks, get outside, and breathe in the fresh air. Connect with the person you are aside from being a care partner
- Do activities you love and that help you keep your mind off your role as a care partner
- Get a treatment you love such as a massage or reiki or go to a yoga class, run, or play tennis. Whatever it is, do something that brings you joy every day
- Seek therapy or counseling if you need or want extra support
- Identify the people in your life you can trust and share your experiences with them
- Be open to what may be the next steps for you and your person with Parkinson's… even if it's not what you imagined. One of the most common reasons for nursing home placement for people with Parkinson's is non-remitting psychosis. If it gets too much for you to manage it on your own, consider potential arrangements that would be best and safest for everyone
- Keep an open line of communication with your person's with Parkinson's care team, and don't be afraid to ask for information, help, or resources

If your loved one is living with Parkinson's disease psychosis, work closely with their movement disorder specialist to assess the situation and create a treatment plan that's right for your person and you. No two people experience Parkinson's disease psychosis in the same way, so it's critical to understand and evaluate all your potential options.

I NO LONGER FEEL LIKE I CAN SUPPORT MY PERSON WITH PARKINSON'S WITHOUT ADDITIONAL ASSISTANCE. WHERE CAN I GO FOR HELP?

As we continually emphasize, you do not have to do everything alone. There are several ways to find help, and one is finding a dedicated caregiver. Professional caregivers often help during the advanced stages of the journey. As your person's Parkinson's progresses, they may experience increasing motor symptoms, and caregivers may need to assist with walking, transfers (in and out of a chair, the shower or bathtub, and bed), food preparation, toileting, bathing routines, and more.

As we have stressed, communication with your person with Parkinson's and the rest of their care team is a critical part of the journey. Do not wait until Parkinson's has progressed to a late stage to discuss caregiving, in-home care, or assisted-living options. Your loved one's physicians can help by discussing the natural progression of Parkinson's and letting you know where your loved one is in the process. This can help you and your support team anticipate and recognize worsening symptoms that are unlikely to improve with medication therapy. This knowledge will prepare you to take appropriate steps when care needs increase.

If hiring an in-home caregiver is the right step for your situation, ask others on your care team, such as your physicians or medical group, for recommendations. Many county websites have a department of health and human services or department of aging that lists providers, and religious organizations may have affiliated or referred agencies. (You might begin with a search for the 211 information for your state. For example, 211Colorado.org connects people to vital resources across the state. Type in your state and 211 to find resources in your state.) You can also reach out to others in your Parkinson's support group for recommendations or organizations like the National Association of Area Agencies on Aging. In Chapter 15 of our *Every Victory Counts* **manual** and online on our *Every Victory Counts* **website**, you can find more in-depth information about the types of care settings and how to choose the best one for your person if you decide this is the best path.

Types of Caregivers. Professional caregivers can work inside your home, in an adult daycare center, at an assisted living facility, in a continuing care retirement community, or in a nursing home. These caregivers may include:

- **Non-certified aides:** As the name implies, these professionals work to help people in their homes but do not have healthcare training. Sometimes called "home helpers" or "home companions," they often help with household tasks, though some may be qualified to assist with routine personal care.

- **Certified nurse's aides (CNA)/home health aides (HHA):** These healthcare employees always work under other healthcare professionals' supervision. They have basic training and can assist with mobility, nutrition, toileting, hygiene, and bedside care.

PART THREE: MANAGING THE COMPLICATIONS OF PARKINSON'S

- **Licensed practical nurses (LPN)/licensed vocational nurses (LVN):** These certified professionals provide basic nursing care and must pass state requirements and a national exam. Although they are qualified to perform some procedures, they must work under the supervision of a physician or registered nurse.
- **Registered nurses (RN):** RNs undergo extensive education and must pass a standardized exam to earn their license. They often administer medication, provide treatment, advise patients, supervise other healthcare workers, and perform all aspects of skilled care.

Whether you transition into the role of caregiver or employ professional help from others (or both!), remember that you provide remarkable and meaningful support. Surround yourself with others who can help support you as you support your person with Parkinson's.

Dear Pat,

From the beginning of this Parkinson's journey, we have been partners, care partners. When we married 21+ years ago, we had no idea what challenges and surprises lay ahead. Some of those challenges were doozies; Parkinson's is one of those. You've had to navigate a minefield of uncertainties and challenges while trying to understand changes in my symptoms and mood. I know this has at times been nothing short of maddening, but you've adjusted and pivoted, all the while keeping me on course.

We both love bike riding, but your enthusiasm is hard to beat. This has given us something to love and do together as we both advocate for people with Parkinson's. In so many areas, we have advocated together—you've been right there with me. You've embraced what I have embraced, and your advocacy and support have made a definite difference, not just for me but for so many people in the Parkinson's world. Thank you for being my advocate buddy.

I came up with the motto, "I plan for the future but live for today." I think replacing "I" with "we" defines our relationship much better. So even though we "live for today," I look forward to growing old (but still strong) together and also having tons of fun "today."

Love,
Cidney

MY ROLE AS A PARKINSON'S CARE PARTNER IS THE MOST REWARDING I HAVE EVER HAD. IT IS POSITIVE IN MANY WAYS, BUT IT IS IMPACTING ME IN NEGATIVE WAYS AS WELL. I AM FEELING LONELY, EXHAUSTED, AND UNDERAPPRECIATED. WHAT CAN I DO?

These feelings, very commonly felt by care partners, can stem from a variety of circumstances. Perhaps it's because you have had to take on roles previously performed by your loved one. Perhaps it's because of excessive demand for your time and attention. And perhaps it's because you set unrealistic expectations for yourself and push yourself to do it all.

Here are a few pieces of advice from Elaine Book, a leader in the Parkinson's community and a social worker with 30 years of experience in community and hospital settings:

- You do not have to be everything for your loved one with Parkinson's. Look and ask for help when you need it. Be specific when you reach out for help and let people know what they can do that would be most helpful.

- Think about who you could add to your loved one's care team to help them and you live well. Would it help you both to connect with a physical, occupational, and speech-language therapist? Do you need to explore home-health options? Who could help with your person's most impactful symptoms? Make a list and reach out to members of your support group or community for recommendations about health providers in your area.

- Remember that you and your loved one with Parkinson's are a team. Communicate, communicate, communicate. Let each other know what forms of help would be most beneficial to you and work together to plan a way forward.

WHAT ARE SOME OF THE SIGNS THAT PARKINSON'S IS PROGRESSING TO THE MOST ADVANCED STAGES?

As we've mentioned several times, since Parkinson's is unique to everyone, not everyone will travel a predictable path. In advanced Parkinson's, your person may experience severe and debilitating symptoms. Motor symptoms, such as rigidity, freezing, and slowness of movement, are often visible and difficult to overcome, and your person may begin to experience increasing non-motor symptoms such as dementia, memory problems, Parkinson's disease psychosis, and incontinence. Your person may need constant assistance to perform everyday tasks, and swallowing can become an increasing challenge. While Parkinson's isn't fatal, people with advanced-stage Parkinson's can experience complications that may be life-threatening, including infections, pneumonia, falls, and choking.

PART THREE: MANAGING THE COMPLICATIONS OF PARKINSON'S

"How can I stay positive when facing the advanced stages of Parkinson's?"

By Gail Gitin

Facing the final days and realizing you and your person with Parkinson's have both fought a long, frustrating, and brave fight against an all-powerful foe is a very difficult place to be, even though we all think about this from the first day of diagnosis. But this is the time to say, "We did all we could; there is no more to do." With that, there comes a feeling of relief that after all these years of fear and wondering, you finally know how it will end and that you will survive this worst of days.

HOW CAN I HELP MY PERSON WITH PARKINSON'S AND MYSELF FIND JOY?

One compelling way is to build gratitude into your everyday lives. At its most basic level, gratitude means thankfulness. More specifically, it means a thankful appreciation of something you have received, be that an experience, a gift, a moment. Practicing gratitude regularly can improve your quality of life, your mental and physical health, your relationships, and more.

THE SCIENCE OF HAPPINESS

In the fall of 2020, renowned Yale professor Laurie Santos, PhD, joined us to discuss the "Science of Happiness," the subject of her widely popular university course. Data shows, she said, that embracing gratitude improves your well-being, your cognition, and your willpower.

"The research shows that the simple act of experiencing gratitude can bump up your well-being," Dr. Santos says. "Especially if you do a daily gratitude practice, it can do that in as little as two weeks. And gratitude is yours free of charge. All you have to do is train your attention toward the blessings in life. The research suggests that shifting to things that give you joy, even small pockets of joy, can boost happiness. The smell of your coffee in the morning. The smile of a family member or friend. Those things are there. We just have to train our mindset to see them."

Happiness, therefore, can be strengthened through practices like mindfulness and gratitude. "We think happiness is something we're born with or is about our circumstances, but the data suggests that like all other good things, it's just something we need to work at," Dr. Santos says. "And as you work at it, just like any other habit, it gets easier over time."

DAILY GRATITUDE EXERCISES

To build this habit of gratitude in your own life as a Parkinson's care partner, train yourself to shift your attention to things that bring you joy instead of concerns over which you have no control. One way to get started with this training is to practice what Dr. Santos calls "rewirements" each day to boost your happiness. Call a friend, write a gratitude letter, perform a random act of kindness, or donate your time to a cause. And when you experience things that bring you joy, whether big or small, take the time to savor them and be fully present.

You can also build a gratitude practice into your daily routine by designating specific "gratitude triggers" to remind you to express gratitude.

By building little moments of gratitude into your daily routine, you will begin to see that your world is filled with things to appreciate, and you will see life as a care partner in a much more positive light.

CELEBRATE EVERY VICTORY

Nothing can fully prepare you for your unique path as a care partner, just as nothing can prepare your loved one for their journey with Parkinson's. It helps to remember that it is a journey—for both of you. Care partner and Davis Phinney Foundation Ambassador Pat Donahoo says it best: "It's a process of learning and working together."

Celebrate victories, such as:

- The chances to live with intentionality
- The space to reflect and grow
- An invigorating workout
- The smell of a freshly brewed cup of coffee
- A new art installation at a local museum
- The satisfaction of finishing a good book
- A hug from a partner, child, or friend
- A lesson learned
- The laughter that erupts from deep in your soul
- The joy of accomplishing something you worked hard on

As Davis Phinney says, "Every Victory Counts." As a care partner, you are a living victory for your person with Parkinson's. Remind yourself that you are doing your best and look for moments of victory every day.

Appendix

■ PARKINSON'S HOME SAFETY TIPS

We frequently ask people with Parkinson's, occupational therapists, physical therapists, and care partners what the most instrumental changes people with Parkinson's can make to their home. We have gathered that information and created this checklist as a starting point to help make your home a great place to live comfortably and safely with Parkinson's.

General Safety Guidelines

Implement these updates everywhere in the house.

- ☐ **Decrease clutter.** Place furniture so that you have wide walkways and can easily move around easily. Decreasing clutter in your physical space not only reduces tripping hazards but also helps to reduce mental clutter and distractions, allowing for greater focus and calm.

- ☐ **Install lever handle door knobs** instead of circular knobs for easier opening.

- ☐ **Install grab bars** throughout your home especially near toilets and within showers and tubs. If possible, seek advice from an occupational therapist (OT) on proper placement first.

- ☐ **Make sure chairs in the house are stable,** have arm rests and are the right height so it is easy to stand from a seated position. Your feet should be able to touch the floor, and your knees and hips should be at approximately 90 degree angles. Soft cushions will make it more difficult to stand up from the chair. Firm boat cushions can be helpful to raise the seat if it is too low.

- ☐ **Lock wheelchair or walker wheels** after each use.

- ☐ **Arrange your furniture to avoid multiple turns or maneuvers** to access areas used every day. This is where you are most likely to fall.

- ☐ **Be sure a communication system is in place** that is easily accessible in every room and hallway that you use. This could be a phone, alarm button or medical alert necklace or bracelet. This is important for people who are in the later stages of Parkinson's.

- ☐ **Give 2-3 trusted individuals keys to your home** in case you need them to come by. Let each of them know who is on your trusted list. Compile their contact information and share with the group if they're comfortable with that. You can also use a lockbox and key, garage door remote code, or a smart lock to offer easy access to your home.

- [ ] **Consider a doorbell with a camera view** so you can see who is at the door.
- [ ] **Consider getting a natural gas detector** for your home. This can be life-saving if you have a diminished sense of smell, which is commonly associated with Parkinson's.
- [ ] **Place the File of Life (folife.org) notice outside** your house and on the side of your refrigerator so that first responders can access it quickly and respect your wishes.
- [ ] Consider getting a **service dog** to help you with freezing of gait at home and elsewhere.
- [ ] **Consider in-home exercise equipment** for exercise options in bad weather. Exercise can improve gait, movement, and mental capacity throughout the day—even short bouts of 10-15 minutes can be helpful.
- [ ] **If you exercise at home,** make sure you have plenty of space to do your workouts.
- [ ] **Request a visit from a physical therapist (PT) or occupational therapist (OT)** who knows the ins and out of Parkinson's to address your needs and offer solutions.
- [ ] **Utilize voice activated music devices** (Alexa, Google Home, etc.) to assist with ungluing from a freeze.

Lighting & Electrical Outlets

- [ ] **Place lights so they are easily accessible.**
- [ ] **Make sure hallways and stairways are well-lit** and use extra lighting to **reduce shadows on steps**.
- [ ] **Use contrasting colors** on light switch plates or get lighted switch plates to make finding switches easy in the dark.
- [ ] **Put night lights in hallways** between bedrooms and bathrooms.
- [ ] Get lamps that you can **turn on with one touch or with sound.**
- [ ] **If possible, install all electrical outlets about waist high** so you don't have to bend down to access them. If not practical, use power strips that are placed within easy reach.
- [ ] **Put all electrical, extension cords, and telephone cords out of the flow of foot traffic** to reduce tripping hazards.
- [ ] **Consider use of smart lights** that can be set to turn on/off at specific times of day.

Floors

- ☐ **Consider installing hardwood flooring and tile** throughout your house. **If you redo your floors,** consider flooring that includes horizontal lines or contrasting grout colors to help with freezing.

- ☐ **Change the paint color in rooms to lighter colors.** It can give the illusion of more space and assist with freezing.

- ☐ **Eliminate abrupt changes in surfaces** (i.e. carpet to hardwood) because they can be a tripping hazard.

- ☐ **Ensure there are handrails on both sides of any area with stairs.** Make sure the rails run the full length of the stairs. Use at least one handrail every time you use the stairs

- ☐ **Remove throw rugs** that could get caught in the wheels of walkers or cause a tripping hazard.

Entryway & Stairs

- ☐ **Install light switches (or motion sensors)** at the top and bottom of the stairs and at every entryway.

- ☐ **Avoid distractions on the stairs,** including conversations or carrying multiple items.

- ☐ **Put a piece of easy-to-see tape at the edge of each step** to help with depth perception.

- ☐ **Use painter's tape to mark proper foot placement** for routine tasks or to guide foot placement through doorways and around corners that might otherwise cause freezing.

Bedrooms

- ☐ **Make sure you can touch your feet to the floor** when seated on your bed to make it easier to get in and out.

- ☐ **Consider installing a side rail,** a sturdy bedside table, or a rope above the bed to assist with rolling and getting up.

- ☐ **Put a bedside commode** next to the bed. This is ideal if you struggle to move easily upon waking.

- ☐ **Always have a bottle of water at the bedside** to assist in raising your blood pressure in the morning if needed.

- ☐ **Securely place blocks, bricks, or other objects under the bed to slightly elevate the head of the bed** and decrease the angle necessary to get out of the bed. This potentially decreases large drops in blood pressure with change in position from supine to sitting if you have neurogenic orthostatic hypotension (nOH).

APPENDIX

☐ **If you have REM Sleep Behavior Disorder,** reduce safety hazards (secure bedside lamps, lock up any weapons, remove clutter) in case you act your dreams out at night or fall out of bed. If you have a spouse or partner, consider sleeping in separate beds.

☐ **Use a motion sensor connected to a light or audible alarm** to notify your spouse or partner if you get up in the middle of the night.

☐ **Consider using a satin sheet for your bottom sheet** to make it easier to roll over.

☐ **Use loose and light sheets** and plan to layer them so you can adjust for comfort relative to the temperature. Also, consider using a single down comforter when it's cold to reduce the chance of getting caught up in multiple sheets. Given this possibility, avoid heated blankets.

☐ **Place a flashlight in the nightstand** or within easy reach in case your power goes out.

☐ **Keep a telephone within easy reach of the bed.**

Bathrooms

☐ **Install grab bars** near the toilet, tub and in the shower. If possible, get help from a PT or OT on proper placement.

☐ **Ensure your toilet is at comfort height** to make it easier to get up and down. You can get a riser if you don't want to replace your toilet.

☐ **Install a stable, purpose-made seat or bench** in your shower. Shower chairs and tub benches can be purchased with arms to increase safety when going from sit/stand.

☐ Make sure all bathtubs, showers floors and exits from shower **are non-slip**. Use aqua socks in public showers.

☐ **Install faucets that turn on and off with one touch.**

☐ **Make sure water temperature** is consistent and not too hot.

☐ **Make sure there is a phone or life alert button** within easy reach of the shower, tub, and toilet in case of an emergency. Better yet, consider using a **waterproof med alert device** such as Revolar in the shower or tub.

Kitchen

☐ **Install faucets that turn on and off with one touch** and can do hot/cold with one hand.

☐ **Consider appliances** that automatically turn off after a certain length of time in case you forget.

- [ ] **Put frequently used items in easy to access locations** so you don't have to bend or reach to get them. No step stools or ladders!

- [ ] **Create prep stations** with all of the supplies for a task within easy reach of the work space (i.e., a coffee station).

- [ ] **Consider trading your ceramic and glass dishes for those made with melamine,** a more durable substance that rarely breaks when dropped.

- [ ] **Swap out large trash cans for smaller ones** or ones with wheels to make it easier to take out the trash.

- [ ] **Try "flicking fingers" periodically** to help with tremor when performing kitchen tasks and eating.

- [ ] **Purchase convenience foods that are pre-cut and washed** to save time and limit the need to use sharp knives.

- [ ] **Make opening jars easier** by using a one-touch, automatic jar opener.

- [ ] **Use non-slip rubber matting** to stabilize cutting boards, mixing bowls or dinnerware.

- [ ] **Weighted utensils and/or utensils with thicker handles** can be helpful for people experiencing tremors.

- [ ] **Place a reacher/grabber** in multiple rooms to assist with grabbing things off the floor that may have fallen. Consider use of a dressing stick, sock aid, long handled shoe horn or long handled sponge to assist with activities of daily living.

APPENDIX

■ PARKINSON'S CARE PARTNERS: REWRITING THE RULEBOOK

This Rulebook is a collaboration between Connie Carpenter Phinney and the Davis Phinney Foundation. It is based on Connie's talk of the same name, Rewriting the Rulebook. You can get your complimentary copy of the illustrated guide at at ⌕ **davisphinneyfoundation.org/parkinsons-care-partner-rulebook**.

RULEBOOK GUIDELINES

Use these guidelines to develop your own rulebook for living well with Parkinson's.

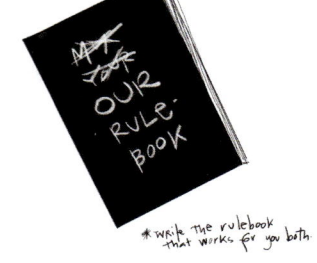

1. **Rule number one is to write your own rulebook!** Parkinson's affects everyone differently as it progresses. What works for another care partner may not work for you. Be smart, observant, and stay informed.

2. **A carefully crafted set of rules** empowers you to achieve optimal health and well-being for you and your person with Parkinson's. When you establish rules, you create a set of communication tools that you can build on to live well now and reference in the future.

3. **Your rulebook should be rooted in knowledge, rely on good manners, and command respect.** You and your person with Parkinson's will travel this path more gracefully when you act with a foundation of knowledge, have faith in each other, and are willing to hold each other accountable. Mind your manners: remember, "please" and "thank you" go a long way.

4. **Your rulebook should be dynamic** and evolve over time as your person with Parkinson's progresses or you experience your own changes in lifestyle or circumstance. Revise existing rules and adapt as needed.

5. **Rules work when they are practical** and encourage mutual caring. Do your best to take care of each other.

BENEFITS OF A RULE BOOK

1. Your rulebook allows you to reset your relationship with your person with Parkinson's. This is pivotal. For example, if your person with Parkinson's is your parent, you may have to overrule decisions they would usually have made. The same may be true of a spouse. Dynamics will shift over time.

2. Rules allow you to define decision-making and focus

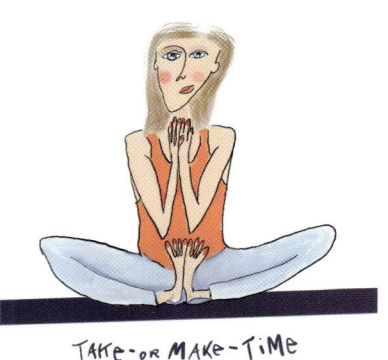

on what matters most: the health, safety, and well-being of you and your person with Parkinson's.

3. Rules help you identify and clarify challenges, wishes, and expectations. When in doubt, use a journal to write out your thoughts and ideas to see what bubbles to the surface. Trust yourself and your instincts.

4. Rules may help you avoid feelings like anger or guilt, which often arise out of lack of clarity.

5. And remember: you are doing the best you can.

RULES FOR YOURSELF

1. **It is fair to acknowledge that you dislike or even hate Parkinson's.** You will experience many feelings after diagnosis and as Parkinson's progresses. Make space to name and feel what you feel. This may include a sense of loss, sadness, anger, and frustration. It is natural to grieve for what could have been after the initial diagnosis and to grieve for what has been lost as Parkinson's advances. Instead of ignoring or putting these strong feelings aside, learn to recognize and soften them to help you live well today. If possible, try to talk it out with a trusted friend, chaplain, or therapist.

2. **Learn to separate the disease from the person living with Parkinson's.** This enables you to be more empathetic. Know, too, that it can be hard to separate the symptoms associated with Parkinson's from the side effects of the medications, so stay informed. Ask your doctor about medication side effects and how changes in dosages may change the severity of side effects, including mood swings. Understand how ON/OFF times and fatigue may also change the behavior of a person living with Parkinson's.

3. **Put your health first**. Many care partners neglect their own health and well-being as they focus so much on the health and well-being of their person with Parkinson's. You won't be able to best care for your person unless you are healthy, too. Schedule time to exercise, see friends, and attend your own doctor appointments. Note that if you are still working, you need this added time even more.

4. **Seek support from other care partners.** You are not alone. Much of what you are experiencing is shared by others, so do try to reach out and connect with care partners who are going through many of the same things. Check out a care partner support group online or nearby. If you don't have one, think about organizing one. Join us for our monthly Care Partner Meetup by registering here: **dpf.org/care-partner-meetup**. Many of our meetups are available on our YouTube channel, and all are discussed in our monthly blog post about the meetup.

5. **Ask for help.** Know that you can't do everything or control all aspects of your person's care. Be honest about what you can and can't do. Ask for help to complete

the tasks you can't do from willing friends and family members. Identify simple tasks that another person can easily do for you. This can lighten your load. And when possible, ask your person with Parkinson's to assist.

6. **Teach your person with Parkinson's to accept help from others.** If you have learned to ask for help early, you'll know who to rely on in a time of need and your person will know how to receive the care of another. For example, designate a friend who can take your person with Parkinson's to physical therapy, take them to exercise, or simply sit with them while you get out.

7. What is important to you and what rules apply?

_____
_____
_____

SAFETY FIRST

Your primary job as a care partner is to ensure your person living with Parkinson's is safe. If your person is doing something that endangers their health and well-being, communicate the threat to their safety and take action to mitigate the danger. Anticipate potential dangers to yourself (like giving yourself space if your person trips often). Be vigilant. Part of making this work is setting the expectation ahead of time that you are the boss and know what is best when it comes to safety.

1. Complete the Parkinson's Home Safety Checklist from the Davis Phinney Foundation. You can order it online at dpf.org/home-safety. Here are some highlights:
   a. Declutter (visually and physically)
   b. Remove tripping hazards (e.g., area rugs)
   c. Minimize "fall" risks (e.g., remove extension cords)
   d. Remove easy access to ladders or stools
   e. Maximize support systems (e.g., grab bars)

2. **Sleep safely.** Between one-third and one-half of people with Parkinson's report REM sleep behavior disorder (RBD) symptoms. A person with RBD acts out vivid dreams in different ways. They may talk in their sleep, jump from the bed, kick or punch a sleep partner, and all of these things happen while they are unaware of their actions. Since RBD can be physically harmful, it's essential to seek a solution. Talk to your doctor about medications and consider adjusting sleep arrangements and rearranging furniture. It may be necessary to get separate beds or sleep in separate rooms.

3. **Are you or others uncomfortable driving with your person with Parkinson's?** If you are, or if you have any doubt about their ability to drive safely, get them tested.

A certified driving rehabilitation specialist (CDRS) can give your person with Parkinson's a comprehensive driving assessment. Following the assessment, the CDRS may provide aides to help your person with Parkinson's drive better or offer restrictions on their driving (e.g., no night driving). These specialists can also help by taking the difficult decision of when to retire from driving out of your hands, helping you avoid highly charged conversations, blame, and guilt.

4. **Get a disabled parking pass.** A disabled parking pass not only provides closer access to your destination, it also typically provides access to larger parking spaces and, therefore, to easier access in and out of the vehicle. This is a simple process arranged through your primary care doctor or neurology office. Get a pass before you need it, and be sure to use it.

5. **Add your own rules around safety and comfort:**

_____
_____
_____

COMMUNICATING WITH YOUR PERSON WITH PARKINSON'S

1. **Create a decision-making framework that works.** Identify what decisions can be made by the person with Parkinson's alone, what decisions you both can weigh in on, and the rarer instances where you can overrule the person with Parkinson's decision as a care partner. For example, if their behavior is threatening their safety or another's safety, you will need to step in. Discussing this ahead of time and taking notes may help if the conversation becomes heated.

2. **Plan ahead for difficult conversations.** People with Parkinson's experience behavior and mood changes throughout the day due to medication side effects, ON/OFF times, fatigue, and various other Parkinson's symptoms. Difficult conversations that may require increased concentration or involve heightened feelings may also escalate the severity of symptoms. Plan ahead to have difficult conversations during a person's ON time or ask them when it is best to talk. Also, be sure to schedule conversations when you are more likely to be patient and will take the time to not only listen, but also to let the person with Parkinson's be heard. Remember, this is a two-way street, but you are in the driver's seat.

3. **Enable your person with Parkinson's.** Tasks help your person with Parkinson's feel and be useful, maintain their independence, and demonstrate their central role in the household. Give them tasks and hold them accountable. Try not to nag. Instead, let your person with Parkinson's get the tasks done at their own pace. For example, it might take Scott twice as long as it takes you to do the dishes—and his dishes may not be as clean as yours—but by doing the dishes, Scott proves to himself—and to you—that he is a contributing member of the household.

APPENDIX

4. **Show compassion.** Symptoms of Parkinson's and side effects of medication can often be a cause of frustration, confusion, and anger, but getting mad will only exacerbate the situation. In most instances, it's best to pause and take a step back. Practicing compassion and patience will be a more productive use of your time and energy and leave you feeling less frustrated.

5. **Add your own rules here or suggested topics to cover or things that are left unsaid:**
   _____
   _____
   _____

COMMUNICATING WITH YOUR DOCTOR

1. **Try to never let your person with Parkinson's go to their doctor appointments alone.** They don't tend to report symptoms fully or represent their needs accurately. Your voice and input are invaluable. A 2010 study found that out of 242 people living with Parkinson's, between 31.8% and 65.2% had undeclared non-motor symptoms. It is well known that patients tend to "spark up" for the doctor, and while your doctor knows and expects this, it's important for you to be able to advocate for him/her by offering your observations to doctors (which may contradict what your person with Parkinson's is saying), asking questions, and providing a second pair of ears to listen to what the doctor has to say.

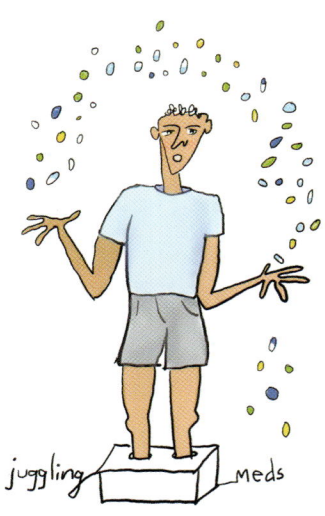
juggling meds

2. **Record the conversation with your doctor.** Have you ever left the doctor's office to find out that your person with Parkinson's heard the doctor say one thing while you heard something different? Rather than argue about what was said and who heard it correctly, if you record the conversations, you can just refer to. A voice recording also frees you from having to take notes while trying to engage with the doctor. Most smartphones have a recording system readily available that you can download and use for free. Be sure to check that it's recording and be sure to "save" the conversation. If you use an app like Otter.ai, it will also provide a transcript which might be especially helpful to share with friends and family to help keep them in the loop. Be sure to ask permission before recording your conversation with a doctor.

3. **Be informed about medication.** Know the side effects (there can be many). Understand dosage and timing. Ask what happens if your person with Parkinson's accidentally misses a dose. Understand ON and OFF times and how they will change your person with Parkinson's mood and behavior. If you don't know if it's a side effect

or if it's the medicine that is causing bizarre behaviors, call your doctor's office. And always be sure to inform your doctor or pharmacist about other medications to be sure they are not contraindicated.

4. **See a movement disorder specialist at least once a year.** A neurologist is a medical doctor who specializes in conditions of the nervous system. A movement disorder specialist is a neurologist with additional training in movement disorders, including Parkinson's. Movement disorder specialists are more familiar with current Parkinson's research and treatment options. It's worth it! Even if you have to fly and arrange travel stays to attend an appointment. The potential improvement in overall care is almost always worth the time, expense, and effort. This also applies for changing doctors, because, over time, you may find your doctor isn't listening as well as he/she should. This might feel risky, but it could also have a huge upside for you both.

5. **Get a signed HIPAA-release from your person with Parkinson's, and make copies of it.** Healthcare providers cannot release health information to you unless you have signed legal documents stating they can release it to you. If your person objects, let them know how important this is for you and ultimately for them. If needed, discuss the reasons with your doctor. They will understand and hopefully help advocate for you. Other legal documents like a durable medical power of attorney are also important as well as discussing your goals for care for the short and long-term. When possible, get everything in writing.

6. **Make a list of documents you currently have and those you will need:**

    _____
    _____
    _____
    _____

7. **Make a separate list of your concerns that haven't been voiced:**

    _____
    _____
    _____
    _____

COMMUNICATING WITH FRIENDS AND LOVED ONES

1. **Be social.** Parkinson's can be isolating, and isolation is bad for your health. Some research suggests it is even worse than smoking two packs of cigarettes per day. It is important to get out and be social, but doing so can require extra planning and energy.

2. **Set boundaries for social events as needed.** Learn when to say no, but don't be afraid to say yes. For example, you might say, "We often find we are too tired to go out in the evening, but we are happy to have you over to our house for a potluck. Please arrive on time and stay no longer than 2 hours."

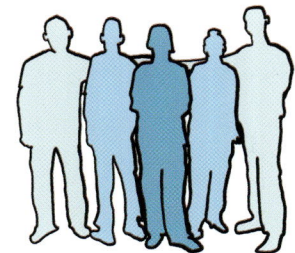

3. **Suggest specific things people can do for you.** People want to help, but they don't always know how. Suggest specific things they can do like, "Can you drop off muffins Tuesday around 10:00 AM and check on Diane?" Or, "Can you sit with Fred while I go to my class?"

4. **Redirect unwanted advice to suggestions for desired help.** Sometimes a loved one's help or advice can feel like a judgment. Learn to communicate when their feedback is unwelcome and then ask them for help in an area you may need it. For example, "Thanks for taking the time to talk to me about exercise and diet, but I have that handled. What I could really use your help with is transportation to his Pedaling for Parkinson's class every Tuesday."

5. **Communicate about expected ON/OFF periods** and ensure phone calls, visits, and other events are scheduled appropriately. Your loved ones often are more concerned about the quality of time you spend together than the quantity. Most will try to accommodate your schedule to ensure you have the best quality time with them while talking, video calling, or visiting.

6. **Make a list of close friends or family you can rely on.**
   Make notes or add your own rules here: _____
   _____
   _____
   _____

7. **What can you do to feel more at ease?**
   Write it down—including how you could make it happen!
   _____
   _____
   _____
   _____

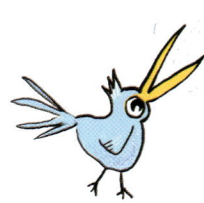

INDEX

A
Aaron Haug 58
Advance Directives 51, 74
Allan Cole 56
Amanda Craig 86
Angela Robb 44
Anxiety 13, 18, 21, 29, 36, 40, 42, 47, 57, 65, 78, 81
Apathy 13, 21, 47, 54, 65, 88

B
Balance 8, 22, 29, 30, 35, 59, 60, 61, 63, 79, 80, 84, 85, 86, 87
Burnout 9, 18, 23, 24, 36, 42, 44, 60

C
Career 19, 32, 79, 80
Caregiver 7, 11, 23, 46, 89, 97, 98
Care Team 8, 11, 12, 14, 15, 18, 21, 30, 41, 43, 51, 61, 65, 77, 84, 85, 91, 96, 97, 99
Cherian Karunapuzha 91
Cognition 28, 89, 100
Cognitive Behavior Therapists 18
Community 7, 9, 12, 15, 16, 18, 19, 22, 24, 36, 40, 43, 46, 50, 52, 54, 55, 63, 64, 69, 78, 83, 84, 85, 88, 92, 97, 99
Connie Carpenter Phinney 7, 28, 32, 108
Coping 16, 19, 31, 35, 38, 40, 79
Counseling 16, 18, 19, 37, 65, 68, 69, 95, 96

D
Delusions 42, 91, 94, 95
Dementia 89, 91, 99
Depression 13, 18, 21, 36, 52, 65, 78, 79, 85, 88
Dopamine 65, 66, 67, 68, 69, 72, 73, 84, 89
Driving 61, 80, 81

E
Exercise 17, 18, 20, 23, 26, 27, 46, 47, 48, 50, 51, 52, 53, 54, 55, 56, 57, 60, 64, 77, 86, 87

F
Falls 29, 30, 31, 84, 99
Family Medical Leave Act (FMLA) 79
Financial Planning 57

G
Gratitude 34, 35, 37, 60, 71, 100, 101

H
Hallucinations 40, 42, 48, 67, 83, 91, 92, 93, 94
Home Safety 103

I
Impulse Control Disorders 66, 70
In-home Care 37, 50, 97
Intimacy 36, 65, 66

J
Janis M. Miyasaki 41
Jessica Shurer 35

L
Living Will 51, 74, 75
Long-term Care 76

M
Mark Mapstone 90
Matthew Ater 62
Medication 12, 13, 14, 18, 27, 41, 51, 58, 64, 65, 66, 67, 68, 70, 71, 72, 73, 74, 78, 87, 89, 91, 93, 95, 97, 98
Memory 90
Motor Symptoms 18, 29, 40, 48, 52, 58, 65, 67, 69, 72, 89, 97, 99
Movement Disorder Specialist 12, 14, 42, 56, 70, 74, 87, 88, 92, 96

N
Nancy Bivins 22, 49
Non-motor Symptoms 18, 29, 48, 65, 69, 72, 99

O
Occupational Therapy/Therapist 14, 42, 54, 103

P
Physical Therapy/Therapists 13, 42, 77, 85, 87, 103
Power of Attorney 51, 74, 75
Psychosis 42, 91, 96, 99

R
Roseanne D. Dobkin 78

S
Stages of Parkinson's 8, 29, 30, 67, 73, 77, 83, 91, 100
Swallowing 14, 29, 30, 31, 42, 99

T
Therapy 87

Y
Young Onset Parkinson's (YOPD) 19, 20, 46, 47, 57, 62, 63, 67

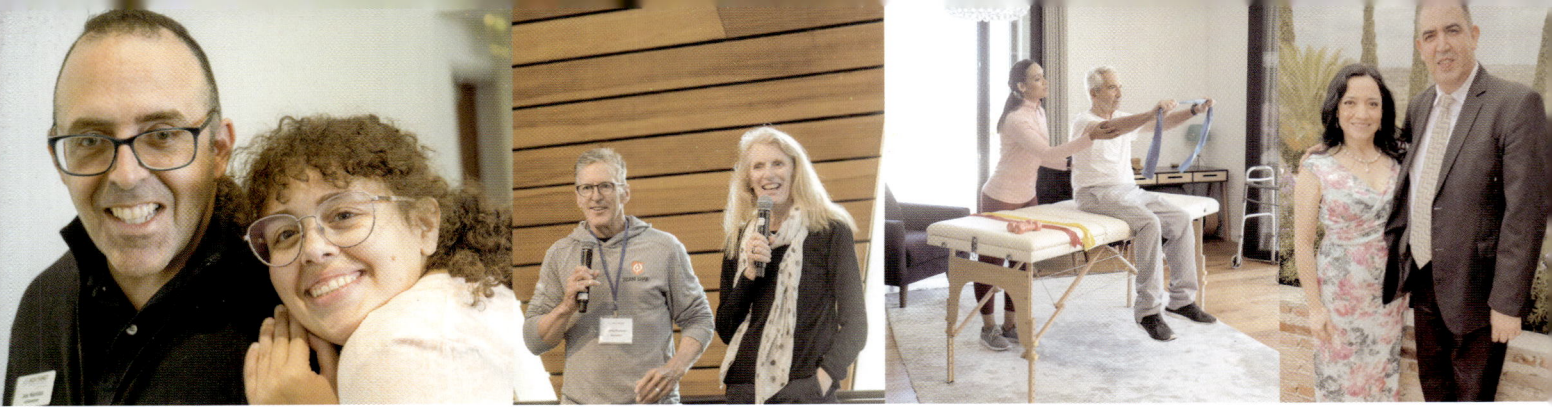

CARE PARTNER TRAINING
A Davis Phinney Foundation Program

Parkinson's Care Partner Training with the Davis Phinney Foundation is a comprehensive educational program led by a movement disorder specialist, clinical social worker, registered dietician, and care partner mentors and created specifically for Parkinson's care partners.

During these sessions, our experts offer education, tools for building self-efficacy, strategies for managing change, and a game plan for navigating the various complications Parkinson's may throw your way.

Visit dpf.org/cp-training to learn more and gain access to pre-recorded sessions which you can watch or listen to whenever it works best for you.

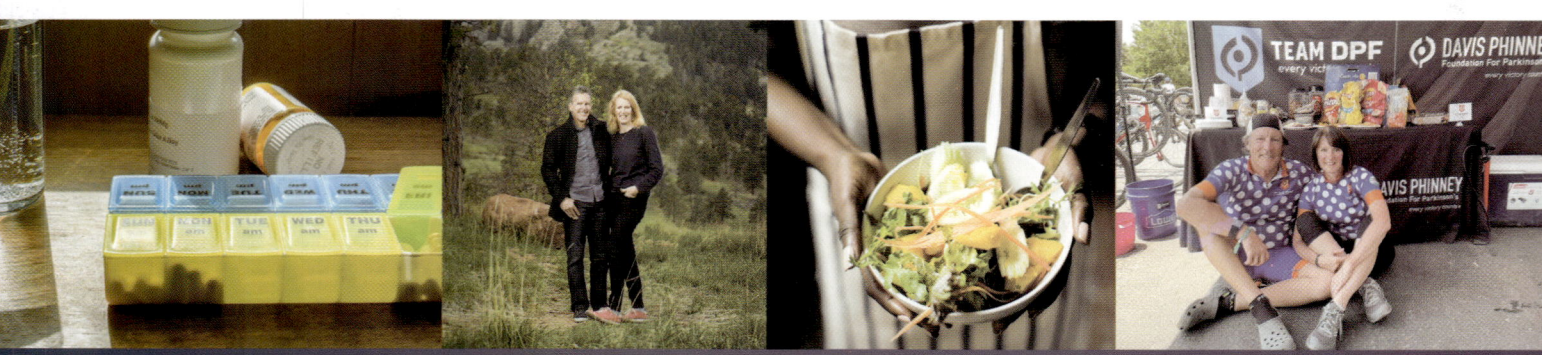

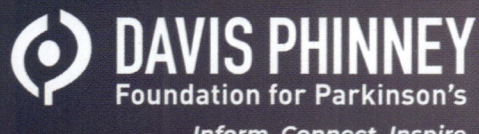

Learn more everything we offer for care partners including additional resources, monthly meetups, and more at dpf.org/resources/im-a-care-partner